MW00848763

Physical Medicine
& Rehabilitation

POCKETPEDIA

Howard Choi, MD
Ross Sugar, MD
David E. Fish, MD, MPH
Matthew Shatzer, DO
Brian Krabak, MD

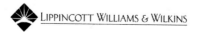

Lippincott Williams & Wilkins

Physical Medicine & Rehabilitation
Pocketpedia

Howard Choi, MD
Fellow, Departments of Physical Medicine & Rehabilitation
Spaulding Rehabilitation Hospital, Harvard Medical School

Fellow, Advanced Spinal Cord Injury Medicine
Boston Veterans Affairs Healthcare System

Postdoctoral Fellow, Department of Neurosurgery, Harvard Medical School
Division of Neurosurgical Research, Boston Veterans Affairs Healthcare System

Ross Sugar, MD
Fellow, Emory University
Georgia Pain Physicians
Pain Management Fellowship

David E. Fish, MD, MPH
Staff Physiatrist
University of California Los Angeles Spine Center

Assistant Professor, Department of Orthopaedics
University of California Los Angeles School of Medicine

Matthew Shatzer, DO
Fellow, Spinal Cord Injury
Kessler Institute for Rehabilitation
Department of Physical Medicine & Rehabilitation
University of Medicine and Dentistry of New Jersey Medical School

Brian Krabak, MD
Assistant Professor and Associate Program Director
Department of Physical Medicine & Rehabilitation
Johns Hopkins University School of Medicine

Assistant Professor
Division of Sports Medicine, Department of Orthopedics
Johns Hopkins University School of Medicine

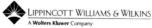

LIPPINCOTT WILLIAMS & WILKINS
A **Wolters Kluwer** Company

Philadelphia · Baltimore · New York · London
Buenos Aires · Hong Kong · Sydney · Tokyo

Executive Editor: Robert Hurley
Developmental Editor: Eileen Wolfberg
Production Editor: Christiana Sahl
Manufacturing Manager: Colin Warnock
Printer: Victor Graphics

© 2003 by LIPPINCOTT WILLIAMS & WILKINS
530 Walnut Street
Philadelphia, PA 19106 USA

Printed in the United States of America

Library of Congress Cataloging-in-Publication Data

ISBN 10: 0-7817-4433-4
ISBN 13: 978-0-7817-4433-1

Care has been taken to confirm the accuracy of the information presented
and to describe generally accepted practices. However, the authors and
publisher are not responsible for errors or omissions or for any consequences
from application of the information in this book and make no warranty,
expressed or implied, with respect to the currency, completeness, or accuracy
of the contents of the publication. Application of this information in a particular
situation remains the professional responsibility of the practitioner.

The authors, consultants, and publisher have exerted every effort to ensure
that drug selection and dosage set forth in this text are in accordance with
current recommendations and practice at the time of publication. However, in
view of ongoing research, changes in government regulations, and the constant
flow of information relating to drug therapy and drug reactions, the reader is
urged to check the package insert for each drug for any change in indications
and dosage and for added warnings and precautions. This is particularly
important when the recommended agent is a new or infrequently employed
drug.

Some drugs and medical devices presented in this publication have Food
and Drug Administration (FDA) clearance for limited use in restricted research
settings. It is the responsibility of health care providers to ascertain the FDA
status of each drug or device planned for use in their clinical practice.

This project was supported in part by unrestricted educational grants from
Pharmacia, Inc., Merck, Inc., and Allergan, Inc. All content, however, has
been exclusively determined by the authors. Common commercial products
are mentioned for informational purposes only; no endorsements are
necessarily implied. Pharmaceutical agent trade names are the property of
the respective manufacturers.

All authors' and consultants' royalties will be donated to non-profit
charitable organizations.

10 9 8 7

TABLE OF CONTENTS

FOREWORD

One of the charges to a program director is to instill in his/her residents the concepts of self-learning and continuing professional development. Recognition of an educational need and accepting the challenge to meet that need are exceptional ways of demonstrating these concepts.

What you have in front of you is a compilation of charts, diagrams, lecture handouts, and other miscellena relevant to the study and practice of PM&R, collected by (former) residents of the Sinai Hospital-Johns Hopkins Training Program*. The intent of this handbook is to provide an accessible and genuinely portable functional formulary for PM&R. This book does not pretend to be comprehensive, nor does it purport to replace the standard PM&R textbooks. There are a multitude of more appropriate sources better suited for those tasks.

Although physicians in training in PM&R are the primary targeted audience of this book, the material in this book is not incompatible with the needs of many other professionals in rehabilitation. I hope that many of you find this little handbook useful.

Gerald Felsenthal MD

GERALD FELSENTHAL, MD
Former Chairman (Retired), Department of
Physical Medicine & Rehabilitation, Sinai Hospital
of Baltimore; Former Program Director,
Sinai Hospital-Johns Hopkins University
School of Medicine Residency Training Program
in Physical Medicine & Rehabilitation

*Drs. Choi, Sugar, Fish, and Shatzer are former residents of the Sinai-Hopkins training program.

INTRODUCTION

The authors would like to express their sincere and deep gratitude for your interest in this handbook. We hope that it serves your needs well. We aspire to make future editions of Pocketpedia as useful to as many of you as possible. If you have any commentary or constructive criticism, please do not hesitate to forward it to howard_choi@hms.harvard.edu.

Again, thanks for your interest in this book, and may your future in Physical Medicine & Rehabilitation be a prosperous one!

Sincerely,
The Authors
September 2, 2002

CONSULTANTS

DAVID T. BURKE, MD, MA
Director, TBI Rehabilitation Program
Spaulding Rehabilitation Hospital
Assistant Professor and Program Director,
Department of Physical Medicine &
Rehabilitation
Harvard Medical School

STEVEN KIRSHBLUM, MD
Director, SCI Services and Ventilator
Dependent Program
Associate Director, Kessler Institute
for Rehabilitation
Associate Professor, Department of
Physical Medicine & Rehabilitation,
University of Medicine and Dentistry-
New Jersey Medical School

ROLAND R. LEE, MD
Associate Professor of Radiology,
University of New Mexico, and
VA Medical Center, Albuquerque
(Formerly, Assistant Professor of
Radiology [Neuroradiology] at
Johns Hopkins University
School of Medicine,
Director of Spine Imaging and
Associate Director of MRI,
Johns Hopkins Hospital)

DAWN LUCIER, PT
Senior Neuro-Physical Therapist
Spaulding Rehabilitation Hospital

ACKNOWLEDGMENTS

The authors would like to express their gratitude to the following individuals for their suggestions, contributions, and/or support for this project (in alphabetical order):

Carol Anders (Sinai Hospital of Baltimore)
Isabel Borras, MD (Sinai Hospital of Baltimore)
Yuemei Corliss, PhD (Allergan, Inc.)
Timothy Dillingham, MD (Johns Hopkins University School of Medicine)
Robert Hurley (Lippincott Williams & Wilkins)
Mary Macy, MD (U.S. Navy, Great Lakes Naval Hospital)
Frank Pidcock, MD (Johns Hopkins University School of Medicine)
Christiana Sahl (Lippincott Williams & Wilkins)
Eileen Wolfberg (Lippincott Williams & Wilkins)
Ellen Zhan, MD (Boston VA Healthcare System)

ABBREVIATIONS AND NOTES REGARDING THE TEXT

Due to considerable space constraints, some unconventional methods were employed to maximize the limited space available. These include: 1) the omission of the phrase "with the permission of the publisher" in some captions (all tables and figures *are* being used with permission of the respective publishers); 2) the listing of only the first author when citing most references (again, severe space constraints have precluded the use of the phrase "et al." in all instances; readers are advised to review the original work for the other authors); 3) the use of non-standardized but commonly used shorthand such as "pt" or "pts" for "patient(s)" and "tx" for "treatment"; included below are some of the abbreviations used in this text.

AC	acromioclavicular	LEx	lower limb/extremity
ACCP	American Coll. of Chest Physicians	LMN	lower motor neuron
		LOC	loss of consciousness
ACL	anterior cruciate ligament	LS	lumbosacral
ADF	ankle dorsiflexion	MCL	medial collateral ligament
ADLs	activities of daily living	MCP	metacarpophalangeal
ADM	abductor digiti minimi	MG	myasthenia gravis
ADQ	abductor digiti quinti plantae	MET	metabolic equivalent
AFO	ankle foot orthosis	MS	multiple sclerosis
AH	abductor hallucis	MTP	metatarsophalangeal
ALS	amyotrophic lateral sclerosis	MUAP	motor unit action potential
APB	abductor pollicis brevis	MVA	motor vehicle accident
APF	ankle plantarflexion	NCS	nerve conduction study
APL	abductor pollicis longus	NCV	nerve conduction velocity
AROM	active range of motion	NIDRR	National Institute on Disability and Rehabilitation Research
ASIA	American Spinal Injury Assoc.		
AVN	avascular necrosis		
b/l	bilateral	NMJ	neuromuscular junction
BKA	below knee amputation	N/V	nausea/vomiting
BMI	body mass index	OOB	out of bed
CMAP	compound motor action potential	ORIF	open reduction internal fixation
CMC	carpometacarpal	PCL	posterior cruciate ligament
COG	center of gravity	PF	plantarflexion
CPM	continuous passive motion	PIP	proximal interphalangeal
CWS	comfortable walking speed	POD	post-operative day
DF	dorsiflexion	PROM	passive range of motion
DIP	distal interphalangeal	PSW	positive sharp wave
DRG	dorsal root ganglion	PT	physical therapy
DTR	deep tendon reflex	PTB	patellar tendon bearing
dx	diagnosis	PWB	partial weight-bearing
ECRB	extensor carpi radialis brevis	RCT	randomized controlled trial
EDC	extensor digitorum communis	RICE	rest, ice, compression, elevation
EHL	extensor hallucis longus		
EMG	electromyography	ROM	range of motion
EPB	extensor pollicis brevis	Rx	prescription
ER	external rotation	SACH	solid ankle cushioned heel
FDI	first dorsal interosseus	SCI	spinal cord injury
FDP	flexor digitorum profundus	SI	sacroiliac
FDS	flexor digitorum superficialis	SNAP	sensory nerve action potential
FES	functional electrical stimulation	SSEP	somatosensory evoked potentials
FPL	flexor pollicis longus		
f/u	follow up	Sx	symptoms
fx	fracture	TBI	traumatic brain injury
GH	glenohumeral	TENS	transcutaneous electrical nerve stimulation
GRF	ground reactive force		
h/a	headache	TFL	tensor fascia latae
HF	hip flexion	THA	total hip arthroplasty
HKAFO	hip knee ankle foot orthosis	TLS	thoracolumbosacral
HMSN	hereditary motor and sensory neuropathy	TMT	tarsometatarsal
		TNF	tumor necrosis factor
HO	heterotopic ossification	TR	transradial
IA	intraarticular	UEx	upper limb/extremity
IP	interphalangeal	UMN	upper motor neuron
IR	internal rotation	US	ultrasound
ITB	iliotibial band	VC	vital capacity
KAFO	knee ankle foot orthosis	VEP	visual evoked potentials
KF	knee flexion	VMO	vastus medialis obliquus
KO	knee orthosis	WB	weight-bearing
LBP	low back pain	WBAT	weight-bearing as tolerated
LEMS	Lambert-Eaton myasthenic synd	WC	wheelchair

I. MUSCULOSKELETAL/SPORTS/ORTHOPEDICS

A. Limb Joint Primary Movers

Motion (ROM in degrees)	Muscles	Nerves	Roots
shoulder flexion (180)	anterior deltoid coracobrachialis	axillary musculocutaneous	**C5,C6** **C6,C7**
shoulder extension (45)	latissimus dorsi teres major posterior deltoid	thoracodorsal inferior subscapular axillary	**C6,C7,C8** C5,**C6,C7** **C5,C6**
shoulder abduction (180)	middle deltoid supraspinatus	axillary suprascapular	**C5,C6** **C5,C6**
shoulder adduction (40)	pectoralis major latissimus dorsi	med+lat pectoral thoracodorsal	**C5-T1** **C6,C7,C8**
shoulder ext rotation (90*)	infraspinatus teres minor	suprascapular axillary	**C5,C6** **C5,C6**
shoulder int rotation (80*)	subscapularis pectoralis major latissimus dorsi teres major	sup+inf subscapular med+lat pectoral thoracodorsal inferior subscapular	**C5,C6** **C5-T1** **C6,C7,C8** C5,**C6,C7**
shoulder shrug	trapezius levator scapulae	spinal accessory (**CN XI**) **C3,C4** ± dorsal scapular (C5)	
elbow flexion (150)	biceps brachii brachialis brachioradialis	musculocutaneous musculocutaneous radial	**C5,C6** **C5,C6** **C5,C6**
elbow extension	triceps brachii	radial	C6,**C7,C8**
forearm supination (80)	supinator biceps brachii	posterior interosseous musculocutaneous	C5,**C6**,C7 **C5,C6**
forearm pronation(80)	pronator teres pronator quadratus	median anterior interosseous	**C6,C7** **C8,T1**
wrist flexion (80)	flexor carpi radialis flexor carpi ulnaris	median ulnar	C6,**C7,C8** C7,**C8,T1**
wrist extension (70)	ext carpi rad long ext carpi rad brev ext carpi ulnaris	radial radial posterior interosseous	**C6,C7** **C6,C7** **C7,C8**
MCP flexion (90)	lumbricales dors+palm interossei	median, ulnar ulnar	**C8,T1** **C8,T1**
PIP flexion (100)	flexor digitorum sup flexor digitorum prof	median median, ulnar	C7-T1 C7,**C8,T1**
DIP flexion (90)	flexor digitorum prof	median, ulnar	C7,**C8,T1**
MCP, finger extension	extensor digitorum extensor indicis extensor digiti min	posterior interosseous posterior interosseous posterior interosseous	**C7,C8** **C7,C8** **C7,C8**

Motion	Muscles	Nerves	Roots
finger abduction (20)	dorsal interossei	ulnar	C8,**T1**
	abductor digiti min	ulnar	**C8,T1**
finger adduction	palmar interossei	ulnar	C8,**T1**
thumb flexion	flexor pollicis brevis	median, ulnar	**C8,T1**
	flexor pollicis longus	anterior interosseous	C7,**C8,T1**
thumb extension	extensor pollicis brev	posterior interosseous	**C7,C8**
	extensor pollicis long	posterior interosseous	**C7,C8**
thumb abduction	abd pollicis long	posterior interosseous	**C7,C8**
	abd pollicis brev	median	**C8,T1**
thumb adduction	adductor pollicis	ulnar	**C8,T1**
hip flexion (120)	iliopsoas	femoral	**L2,L3**,L4
hip extension (30)	gluteus maximus	inferior gluteal	**L5,S1**,S2
hip abduction (40)	gluteus medius	superior gluteal	L4,**L5,S1**
	gluteus minimus	superior gluteal	L4,**L5,S1**
hip adduction (20)	adductor longus	obturator	**L2,L3**,L4
	adductor magnus	obturator, sciatic	L2,L3,**L4,** L5,S1
hip external rotation (45)	obturator int+ext	n. obt int, obturator	L3-S2
	quadratus femoris	n. quadratus femoris	**L2,L3**,L4
	piriformis	n. piriformis	**S1**,S2
	sup+inf gemelli	n. obt int, n. quad fem	L4-S2
	glut max (post fibers)	inferior gluteal	**L5,S1**,S2
hip internal rotation (45)	gluteus minimus	superior gluteal	L4,**L5,S1**
	gluteus medius	superior gluteal	L4,**L5,S1**
	tensor fasciae latae	superior gluteal	L4,**L5,S1**
knee flexion (135)	semitendinosus	tibial div. of sciatic	**L5,S1**,S2
	semimembranosus	tibial div. of sciatic	L4,**L5-S2**
	biceps femoris	tib+per div. sciatic	L5,**S1,S2**
knee extension	quadriceps femoris	femoral	**L2,L3,L4**
ankle dorsi-flexion (20)	tibialis anterior	deep peroneal	**L4,L5**,S1
ankle plantar-flexion (45)	gastrocnemius	tibial	L5,**S1**,S2
	soleus	tibial	L5,**S1,S2**
ankle inversion (35)	tibialis posterior	tibial	L4,**L5**,S1
ankle eversion (25)	peroneus longus	superficial peroneal	L4,**L5**,S1
	peroneus brevis	superficial peroneal	L4,**L5,S1**
toe extension	extensor hallucis longus	deep peroneal	L4,**L5**,S1
	extensor digitorum brev	deep peroneal	**L5,S1**

*Shoulder IR/ER varies with elevation of the arm.
For ROM, 0° is anatomic position. Please note that there is no absolute concensus regarding which muscles are the primary movers of joints or for the root innervations of muscles.

4

B. Tx of Selected Musculoskeletal Conditions

1. Upper limb

Acromioclavicular (AC) sprains/tears - AC injuries may be seen with falls on the adducted shoulder. A type I (Rockwood classification) injury is a non-displaced sprain of the AC ligament, manifested by local tenderness w/o anatomic deformity. A

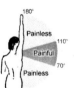

Fig.1

type II injury (see Fig.1) involves an AC tear and coracoclavicular (CC) ligament sprain, but the CC interspace is intact. Tx for type I or II injuries includes an arm sling, ice, analgesics, and progressive ROM exercises. An unstable type II injury may require arm sling use for 2-4wks. Sports activities can be resumed when full painless ROM is achieved and deltoid strength is near-baseline. Type III-VI lesions involve rupture of the AC *and* CC ligaments with varying displacements of the clavicle. These require orthopedic consultation for potential ORIF, although many separations may be followed conservatively with several wks of sling-and-swath immobilization, followed by long-term therapy.

Rotator cuff tendinitis/shoulder impingement syndrome - Predisposing and causative factors include acromion shape and repetitive overhead activities (i.e., throwing, racquet sports, swimming). Pain and aching are often worse at night, and can be aggravated by overhead activities. Shoulder flexion and abduction may be limited.

A *painful arc* may be present at about 70-110° on passive arm abduction. *Neer's test* and *Hawkins test* evaluate for shoulder impingement. In Neer's test, the examiner fixes the scapula with one hand and elevates the subject's arm with the other. Pain indicates a positive test. Hawkins test is done by abducting the subject's arm to 90° with the elbow flexed, then internally rotating the shoulder. Hawkins test can also be done in the scapular plane. In the *drop arm test*, the arm is passively elevated in abduction and the patient is asked to hold the arm in position. Inability to do so may be indicative of a severe or complete tear of the rotator cuff.

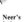

Neer's test

The painful shoulder should initially be *rested* until pain and swelling subside. *Ice* and *NSAIDs* may be helpful. Overhead activities should be avoided. *PT* can institute gentle stretching and strengthening to preserve ROM. A *steroid injection* into the subacromial space may relieve pain if the above measures fail. A repeat injection should be avoided in pts with <2 months of pain relief following the 1st injection.

Exercises should progress until strength and ROM are restored. *Surgery* is an option if several months of conservative tx/steroid injections fail to resolve the sx (or for complete tears). An acromioplasty, the most common procedure, involves acromial shaving to increase the space around the inflamed tendon. The tendon may also be debrided. Several months may be required to regain full strength after surgery.

Fig.1 courtesy of **Rockwood CA**, ed.: *Rockwood & Green's Fxs in Adults*, 3rd ed. JB Lippincott, 1988.

Anterior shoulder dislocation - Anterior dislocations are more common than posterior dislocations. Complications include axillary nerve injury, recurrent dislocations, and rotator cuff tears (especially in older pts). A *Bankart lesion* (left) is an avulsion of the anteroinferior glenoid labrum and capsule from the glenoid rim and is felt to be a primary etiologic factor in recurrent dislocations. A *Hill-Sachs lesion* is a compression fx of the humeral head when the posterolateral aspect of the humeral head compresses against the anterior glenoid rim. Age at initial dislocation is prognostic for recurrence: teens/young adults have significantly higher redislocation rates (said to approach 90%) than older pts (said to be ~10-15% for pts >40y/o).

Various techniques for acute reduction exist, including the modified *Stimson technique*, where the pt lies prone with a wrist weight (i.e., 5-10 lbs) on the affected arm as it hangs over the side of the table. Reduction is achieved over 15-20mins as the shoulder muscles relax.

Early rehabilitation may include icing and sling immobilization for 1-3 wks to allow for healing of the capsule. Maintenance of elbow, wrist and hand ROM is important. Isometric exercises and gentle pendular exercises with the arm in the sling are encouraged, but passive abduction for hygiene is limited to 45° and external rotation is avoided. The duration of sling use may be shortened in older pts due to the higher risk of frozen shoulder. Once the capsule has healed, shoulder ROM and strengthening are progressed. There is some debate regarding the optimal type and timing of surgery after shoulder dislocation and in shoulder instability.

Adhesive capsulitis - A syndrome characterized by a progressive painful loss of passive and active glenohumeral ROM. Abduction and external rotation are most affected; internal rotation is least affected. This condition may be the end result of other conditions that result in prolonged immobility (i.e., bursitis, rotator cuff tendinitis). Treatment can consist of an aggressive ROM program, with NSAIDs and heat modalities to improve tolerance. Other techniques include steroid injections and manipulation under anesthesia. Recovery may take several months to a year.

Bicipital tendinitis - This overuse injury can be associated with overhead activities or sports, and often co-exists with the shoulder impingement syndrome. Examination reveals a tender bicipital groove. *Speed's test* (left) is performed by elevating the subject's arm to 90° with the elbow extended and palm upward, then having the pt attempt forward flexion of the arm against resistance. Pain in the bicipital groove is a positive test. Tx includes NSAIDs, activity modification, and progressive exercise program, which may include the use of modalities such as heat and post-activity icing. Local corticosteroid injection may be used in refractory cases.

Scapular winging - Medial scapular winging is caused by weakness of the serratus anterior (long thoracic n.). It is elicited by having the pt push off against a wall.

Medial Winging   Lateral Winging

Lateral winging is caused by weakness of the trapezius muscle (CN XI) and is elicited by shoulder abduction.

Golfer's elbow (medial epicondylitis) - An overuse syndrome of the tendinous origin of the flexor-pronator mass and MCL of the elbow. The initial tx is *RICE* (relative rest, ice, compression, elevation) and *NSAIDs*. Stretching the elbow during the painful period is important. Once pain and inflammation subside, strengthening exercises are started (important groups include the wrist flexors/ extensors, wrist radial deviators, forearm pronator/supinators, and elbow flexor/extensors). *Injection of local steroids* into the area of max tenderness can be also considered, with care taken not to injure the ulnar n. A *tennis elbow strap* may be helpful.

Tennis elbow (lateral epicondylitis) - An extensor tendinopathy, especially of the *ECRB*. The initial tx is *relative rest, NSAIDs, and heat or cold* modalities. Wrist extensor *stretching* and *strengthening* should be initiated when tolerated. Conservative measures are usually effective, but recurrences are common. A tennis elbow strap worn circumferentially around the forearm just distal to the elbow may be helpful. Modifications to the racquet include a *larger racquet grip and head* and *lessening string tension*. A *corticosteroid injection* into the area of max tenderness may be indicated if conservative tx fails (see p.129). No more than 3 injections should be given at intervals of 5d to 1wk. Surgical fasciotomy or fixation of the conjoined tendon may be considered if the above measures fail.

DeQuervain's disease - A tenosynovitis of the 1st dorsal compartment of the hand, including the APL and EPB tendons. *Finkelstein's test* is positive when pain is elicited in the radial wrist while the wrist is forced into ulnar deviation with the thumb enclosed in a fist. Tx includes *activity modification* and *NSAIDs*, then a *stretching* and *strengthening* program. A *thumb spica splint* with the wrist in neutral and the 1st MCP immobilized (IP joint is free) is helpful in resting the tendons. *Local corticosteroid injections* (max of 3) into the compartment reduce acute pain and inflammation (see p.129). *Surgical decompression* may be curative in severe, refractory cases.

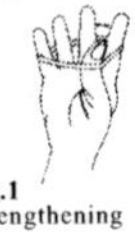

Fig.1
Strengthening

Scaphoid fx (most common carpal bone fx) - Often due to a fall on an outstretched hand. Snuffbox tenderness may be noted. If initial plain films (~3-4 views) are negative, the wrist should be immobilized (short arm cast or splint with thumb spica) and films repeated in ~2wks (some fxs may not be visible until bone has resorbed around the fx line). If repeat films are negative and clinical suspicion persists, CT or MRI can be considered.

Because the main blood supply enters from the distal pole, there is a high incidence of non-union and AVN in waist and proximal pole fxs. Non-displaced fxs should be placed in a *long arm thumb spica cast*. Isometric muscle contractions can be performed in the cast to counter atrophy. Displaced fxs or non-displaced fxs with persistent non-union should be referred for surgical evaluation.

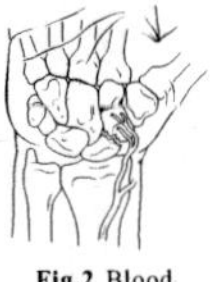

Fig.2 Blood supply of the scaphoid

Fig.1 courtesy of **Rouzier P**: *The Sports Medicine Patient Advisor*. SportsMed Press, 1999.

Trigger finger (digital stenosing tenosynovitis) - Digital tendon sheath inflammation may result in a tendinous knot that gets stuck in the finger pulley system as the finger extends. Pts with DM or RA are particularly at risk of developing trigger finger. *NSAIDs* and *steroid injections* help to reduce inflammation and pain. Use of a *volar static hand splint* that immobilizes the MCP but allows full IP flexion rests the flexor tendons and helps to break the vicious cycle of inflammation and catching. In some cases, surgery may be necessary to release tendons in fingers that are locked in flexion.

2. Lower limb

Trochanteric bursitis - Pain is noted with walking, running, or laying on the involved hip. On exam, point tenderness over greater trochanter is noted. Conservative treatment includes *NSAIDs* and an ITB *stretching* program. A *steroid injection* into the bursa can relieve symptoms in many pts.

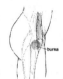

Figure courtesy of **Rouzier** P: *The Sports Medicine Patient Advisor.* SportsMed Press, 1999.

Iliotibial band syndrome - Potential causes include over-training or running over uneven surfaces. Lateral knee pain is noted as the ITB slides over the lateral femoral condyle, especially between 20-30° of flexion. Tenderness over the lateral knee and Gerdy's tubercle may be noted on exam. *Ober's test* may be positive. Rehabilitation should be aimed at *stretching* the ITB, hip flexors, and gluteus maximus. Adductors may be strengthened to counteract the tight ITB.

Fig.1. Hip adduction strengthening with Theraband

Helpful *modalities* include ice, US, and phonophoresis. Foot pronation should be corrected; running only on even surfaces may help. A *steroid injection* into the area of the lateral femoral condyle may relieve pain. Symptoms can generally take 2-6mos to improve.

Right: The Ober test for ITB/TFL contraction. The pt lies on the side with the involved side uppermost. The hip is flexed, then abducted as far as possible while stabilizing the pelvis. Next, the hip is brought into extension and the limb is released. The limb will remain abducted if there is tightness at the ITB or TFL.

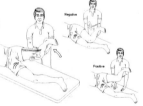

Pes anserine bursitis (bursa under *S*artorius, *G*racilis, semi*T*endinosis, Mnemonic: "*S*ay *G*race before *T*ea") - Pain and tenderness at the insertion of the medial hamstrings at the medial proximal tibia may be noted. The tx should emphasize *stretching* of the medial hamstrings. *Steroid injections* may be very effective. Athletes may wear *protective knee padding*.

Fig.1 courtesy of **Rouzier** P: *The Sports Medicine Patient Advisor.* SportsMed Press, 1999.

Anterior cruciate ligament (ACL) - The ACL proceeds superiorly and posteriorly from its anterior medial tibial attachment to attach to the medial aspect of the lateral femoral condyle. It prevents excessive anterior translation of the tibia and abnormal ER of the tibia on the femur and knee hyperextension. A primary function in the athlete is maintaining joint stability during deceleration.

Fig.1

Injuries may be due to excessive *pivoting* or *cutting* as well as hyperextension, hyperflexion or lateral trauma to the knee. A "pop" is often heard or felt at the time of injury. Immediate swelling and a sense of instability may follow.

The *Lachman test* (**Fig.2**) is done at 20-30° of knee flexion and particularly assesses the posterolateral fibers. Some laxity may be normal, so comparison with the contralateral leg is recommended. Sensitivity is higher than the anterior drawer test (99% vs. 54%)[1]. The *pivot-shift (MacIntosh) test* is performed in the lateral decubitus position with the affected knee extended and the tibia internally rotated. Valgus stress is applied to the knee as it is flexed. A "clunk" felt at 30° of knee flexion is indicative of ACL injury. A *MRI* confirms the dx and may identify other concomitant injuries.

Non-operative rehabilitation of ACL injury should concentrate on proprioceptive training and strengthening of the hamstrings (i.e., TheraBand; see **Fig.3**) to prevent anterior subluxation of the tibia. Terminal range squats to strengthen the quads should be encouraged to prevent patellofemoral pain, a frequent occurrence after ACL tears. Bracing should limit terminal extension and rotation.

The need for *operative tx* depends on the amount of damage, degree of laxity, and is pt-specific as well. A younger, more active pt is more likely to require surgical repair vs. the older, sedentary pt. Post-op rehab can last up to 6-9mos, although the trend is to shorten this time. Pts are typically WBAT with an extension brace immediately after surgery. As with non-operative rehab, the emphasis is on strengthening the hamstrings and proprioceptive training. During the first six weeks, it is important to regain ROM (can be assisted by CPM) and enhance patellar mobility. Intensity and resistance should progressively increase between wks 6-10. By wk 10, there should essentially be no limitation in strengthening.

References: **1**. **Torg JS**: Clinical dx of ACL instability in the athlete. *Am J Sports Med* 1976;4:84-93. **Figs.1,2** courtesy of **Fu F, Stone D**: *Sports Injuries: Mechanisms, Prevention & Treatment.* Williams & Wilkins, 1994. **Fig.3** courtesy of **Rouzier P**: *The Sports Medicine Patient Advisor.* SportsMed Press, 1999.

Posterior cruciate ligament (PCL) - The PCL arises from the posterior intercondylar tibia and extends anteriorly, superiorly, and medially to attach to the medial femoral condyle. It prevents abnormal IR and posterior translation of the tibia on the femur, which aids knee flexion.

Injury of the PCL classically occurs 2° to a MVA when the tibia strikes the dashboard, forcing the tibia posteriorly. Injury also occurs with high valgus stress or when falling on a flexed knee. Swelling is uncommon. Integrity of the PCL can be tested by the *posterior drawer test* and the *sag test*, where the examiner tries to observe a posterior displacement of the tuberosity with the quadriceps relaxed.

Treatment of a mild PCL sprain usually involves quadriceps strengthening without need for bracing. Severe PCL injuries will often need to be repaired arthroscopically.

Figure courtesy of **Fu F, Stone D**: *Sports Injuries: Mechanisms, Prevention & Tx.* Williams & Wilkins, 1994.

Meniscal injury - The menisci increase the contact area between the femur and tibia and can act as "shock absorbers" for the knee.

Transverse ligament
ACL
Medial
Lateral
PCL Ligament of Wrisberg

Mechanisms of injury include excessive rotational stresses, typically the result of twisting a flexed knee. The medial meniscus is more often injured than the lateral.

Knee locking, popping, and/or clicking are characteristic complaints. On exam, an effusion, joint line tenderness, and loss of full knee extension may be noted. *McMurray's test* is performed with pt supine and hip and knee maximally flexed. A valgus-tibial ER force is applied while the knee is extended; a pop or snap suggests a medial meniscus tear. Varus-tibial IR forces are used to evaluate the lateral meniscus. McMurray's test may be poorly tolerated due to pain and is felt by some to be relatively unreliable[1]. Apley's grind test may be positive, but is avoided by some clinicians for fear of aggravating the injury. *MRI* may help confirm the clinical dx and identify other injuries. *Arthroscopy* is the gold standard for dx of a tear.

Tx is dependent on the severity of injury. For the non-surgically treated pt, early management consists of *RICE*, NSAIDs, and hamstring and ITB *stretching*. A joint aspiration is sometimes useful to reduce effusion and relieve pain. *Aquatic exercises* and *canes* can unload the affected meniscus. The intensity can be gradually increased with avoidance of activities involving compressive rotational loading. It may be reasonable to gradually resume sports activities once strength in the affected limb approaches 70-80% of the unaffected limb. Orthopedic referral for possible *arthroscopic surgery* is indicated if the pt is experiencing mechanical symptoms including locking, buckling, or recurrent swelling with pain.

Surgical treatment has been evolving. Total meniscectomy is no longer considered acceptable; efforts are now aimed at preserving as much cartilage as possible in order to prevent degenerative changes. The outer thirds of the menisci are vascular and may be repaired; the inner two-thirds are avascular and may need to be debrided. Following partial meniscectomy, full WB may occur once the pt is pain free. Following meniscal repair, full WB may be delayed for up to 6wks. ROM exercise, stretching, and progressive strengthening of the lower limbs are the mainstays of post-op therapy. Deep squatting is discouraged.

References: **1. Scholten RJ**: The accuracy of physical dx tests for assessing meniscal lesions of the knee: a metaanalysis. *J Fam Pract* 2001;50:955-7. Figure courtesy of **Fu F, Stone D**: *Sports Injuries: Mechanisms, Prevention & Treatment.* Williams & Wilkins, 1994.

10

Patellofemoral pain syndrome - The etiology
is postulated to be a combination of overuse,
muscular imbalance, and/or biomechanical
problems (i.e., pes planus or pes cavus, ↑ Q
angle). Anterior knee pain may occur with
activity and worsen with prolonged
sitting or descending stairs.

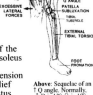

Above: Sequelae of an
↑ Q angle. Normally,
♂ Q is 13°; ♀ is 18°.
Figure courtesy of **Fu**
F. Stone D: *Sports
Injuries: Mechanisms,
Prevention & Tx.*
Williams & Wilkins.

Acute management involves
relative rest, ice, and *NSAIDs.*
Prolonged sitting should be avoided.
The mainstay of rehabilitation is to
address the biomechanical deficits
through a combination of *quadriceps
strengthening exercises* with *stretching* of the
quadriceps, hamstrings, ITB, and gastroc-soleus
complex.

Classically, short arc terminal knee extension
(0-30°) exercises were utilized, with the belief
that they selectively strengthened the vastus
medialis obliquus (VMO). Currently the idea of
VMO selectivity is controversial. In general,
short arc (0-45°) closed kinetic chain leg press
exercises are recommended to strengthen all 4
heads of the quads, which are thought to be
weakened in aggregate. Full-arc and open kinetic chain exercises
should be avoided to reduce symptom aggravation.

Taping the patella so that it tracks properly (*McConnell
technique*) may improve pain symptoms during exercise. *Orthotics*
to correct pes planus or foot pronation and soft braces with patellar
cutouts may provide modest symptomatic relief in appropriate cases.
Occasionally, *electrical stimulation* and *biofeedback* are useful.
Prolonged PT with modalities such as US is generally not helpful or
cost-effective. *Surgery* is rarely necessary and is reserved for
recalcitrant instability or symptomatic malalignment.

Exercise-induced leg pain - Shin splint, a non-specific term, refers to
exercise-induced tibial pain, without evidence of fx on xray. It is
believed to represent periostitis, usually of the posteromedial tibial
border (*medial tibial stress syndrome*). Runners, gymnasts, and
dancers are at risk, with causes including an increase in exercise
intensity, inadequate footwear, hard surface training, or poor
biomechanics. Local pain and tenderness are noted along the distal
1/3 of the tibia. Pain is often quickly relieved by rest, and not
aggravated by passive stretch. Bone scan may be positive in severe
cases. Tx includes rest, NSAIDs, US, peri-activity icing, and
correction of aggravating factors.

Causes of *tibial stress fxs* (TSF) are similar to those of tibial
stress syndrome. Stress fxs are also common in the fibula and the
metatarsals, especially the 2nd metatarsal. Pain is initially exercise-
induced only, but progresses to pain with weight-bearing or even at
rest. There is often exquisite point tenderness along the distal or
middle third of the tibia. X-rays may be negative early, but may show
a clear fx after several wks (i.e., a positive "dreaded black line" on
oblique radiograph, representing an anterior TSF). Bone scans are
more sensitive. TSFs can be treated with *relative rest* (i.e., crutches).
Medial TSFs can be treated with relative rest for 4-6wks, NSAIDs,

and TENS. Anterior TSFs may require several months of rest from sports activities and ongoing conservative tx. Recalcitrant cases may eventually require a bone graft.

In *chronic compartment syndrome of the leg*, pain is felt after a specific period of exercise, and can be associated with parasthesias, numbness, and weakness in the distribution of the nerve within the compartment. EDx studies are usually normal. Resting and post-exercise compartment pressures should be obtained. Resting pressures >30mm Hg, 15sec post-exercise pressures >60mm Hg, or 2min post-exercise pressures >20mmHg are all suggestive of chronic compartment syndrome. An initial conservative approach should include NSAIDs, proper footwear selection and correction of training errors. If symptoms persist 1-2mo after a trial of conservative tx, referral for surgical fasciotomy may be warranted.

Achilles tendinitis - Overuse, overpronation, heel varus deformity, and poor flexibility of the Achilles tendon/gastroc-soleus/hamstrings may be contributing factors. Basketball players may be particularly susceptible due to the frequent jumping. It is also noted in runners who increase their mileage or hill training. Symptoms include pain and swelling in the tendon during and after activities. On exam, there may be swelling, pain on palpation, a palpable nodule, and inability to stand on tiptoes. Chronic tendinitis may result in tendon weakness, potentially leading to rupture.

There is no consensus on optimal mode of treatment, but most rehabilitation will likely begin with the *PRICE* principle (protection, rest, ice, compression, elevation). Modalities, especially *US*, may be helpful. Plantarflexor strengthening is important. *Downhill exercises* should be emphasized; uphill running should be discouraged, especially early in rehab. Heel lifts may provide early relief but may lead to heel cord shortening with prolonged use. A properly fitted shoe, often with a stiff heel counter, is important. Injection of the Achilles tendon is not recommended by many sources due to risk of tendon rupture. For severe or chronic cases, recovery to near-normal strength may take up to 24 months, even with good circulation. Young, active persons with ruptured tendons are usually operated on; casting is an option for older, sedentary persons.

Ankle sprains - Lateral ankle sprains are usually due to inversion of a plantarflexed foot. The anterior talofibular ligament (ATFL) is typically the first structure to be involved. With increasing severity of injury, the calcaneofibular ligament (CFL) may be involved next, followed by the posterior talofibular ligament (PTFL). The anterior drawer test checks ankle ligament stability (displacement ≥5mm is considered positive). The talar tilt test (right) checks the CFL; it is performed by providing an inversion stress on the talus (a positive test is a marked difference, i.e., >10°, in the inversion of the affected vs. the unaffected side). X-rays to check the tibial-fibular syndesmosis may be necessary in the event of severe sprains; these require surgical consultation.

Torn ATFL
Torn CFL

Injuries of the medial (deltoid) ankle ligament due to an eversion injury are less common; an associated proximal fibula fracture (Maisonneuve fx) should be ruled out.

Rehabilitation of ankle sprains involves three phases: *Phase I* normally lasts 1-3 days, until the pt is able to bear weight comfortably. This phase involves the *RICE* principle: rest (i.e., crutches), ice 20mins 3-5×/day, compression with ACE wrap, and elevation of the foot above the heart. Hot showers, EtOH, methylsalicylate counterirritants (i.e., Ben Gay) and other txs that may increase swelling should be avoided during the initial 24hrs. *Phase II* usually lasts days to weeks. The goals in this phase are to restore ROM, strengthen the ankle stabilizers, and stretch/strengthen the Achilles tendon. *Phase III* is initiated when motion is near normal and pain and swelling are almost absent. Re-establishing motor coordination via proprioceptive exercises and endurance training are emphasized, i.e., balance board, running curves (figure-of-8) and zig-zag running.

Return to play recommendations vary. Some recommendations may be as follows: Grade I (no laxity and minimal ligamentous tear): 0-5 days. Grade II (mild to moderate laxity and functional loss): 7-14 days. Grade III (complete ligamentous disruption, cannot bear weight): 21-35 days. Syndesmosis injury: 21-56 days.

Figure courtesy of Fu F, Stone D: *Sports Injuries: Mechanisms, Prevention & Treatment.* Williams & Wilkins, 1994.

Plantar fasciitis - Commonly seen in athletes and in persons whose jobs require a lot of standing or walking. Repetitive microtrauma to the plantar fascia can cause inflammation and pain. Biomechanical issues (i.e., an overpronated foot with increased tension on the fascia) are often at fault. The classic symptoms are heel pain on the first few steps in the morning, or pain that is worse at the beginning of an activity.

The key component of tx is a home exercise program of *routine, daily stretching* of the plantar fascia and Achilles tendon. Pts should be on *relative rest* from walking, running, and jumping and consider switching to activities such as swimming or cycling to allow for the fascia to heal. *Proper footwear* includes well-cushioned soles, possible use of an extra-deep heel pad/cup insert, and avoiding high heels. *Soft medial arch supports* are generally preferable to rigid orthotics, which can exacerbate symptoms. NSAIDs and ice may help decrease inflammation. *Splints* to supply a gentle constant stretch across the sole of the foot at night while sleeping are useful in pts not responding to other measures. Once the pain resolves, pts should only gradually return to increased levels of activity, while continuing their stretching program.

The majority of cases will improve with conservative measures w/in 6-12 weeks, if faithfully followed. In the rare, persistent case, a *local corticosteroid injection* may be considered. A potential complication is necrosis of the fatty pad of the heel, which cannot be easily reversed or treated. Surgical intervention, which consists of a release of the involved fascia from its attachment to the calcaneus, can be considered if all other measures fail, but is necessary in only very rare cases.

Figure courtesy of **Rouzier P**: *The Sports Medicine Patient Advisor.* SportsMed Press, 1999.

C. Sports/Exercise Preparticipation Evaluation (PPE)

1. General guidelines

Questions about personal and family hx of cardiovascular disease are the most important initial component of the H&P. A thorough hx of neurologic or musculoskeletal problems should also be emphasized. Physical exam should emphasize cardiac auscultation with provocative maneuvers to screen for hypertrophic cardiomyopathy (see below), which is the most common cause of sudden death in young male athletes. For most young, asymptomatic persons, screening tests such as electrocardiography, treadmill stress testing and lab tests are not indicated in the absence of symptoms or a significant hx of risk factors[1]. For older asymptomatic persons w/o cardiopulmonary risk factors or known metabolic disease, the American College of Sports Medicine recommends exercise stress testing in men ≥45yrs and women ≥55yrs before starting a vigorous exercise program (≥60% of VO_2 max)[2]. Most older persons can begin a moderate aerobic and resistance training program without stress testing if they begin slowly and gradually increase their level of activity[3].

Reference: **1. Kurowski K, Chandran S**: The preparticipation athletic evaluation. *Am Fam Physician* 2000;61:2683-98. **2. ACSM**: *Guidelines for exercise testing and prescription,* 6th ed. LWW, 2000. **3. Neid RJ**: Promoting and prescribing exercise for the elderly. *Am Fam Physician* 2002;65:419-28.

2. Example of an appropriate preparticipation PE

Exam feature	Comments
Blood pressure	Must be assessed in the context of participant's age, height and gender.
General	Measure for excessive height and observe for evidence of excessive long bone growth that suggests Marfan syndrome
Eyes	Important to detect vision defects that leave one of the eyes with worse than 20/40 corrected vision.
Cardiovascular	Palpate the point of maximal impulse for increased intensity and displacement that suggest hypertrophy or failure, respectively.
	Perform auscultation with the pt supine and again at standing or straining during Valsalva's maneuver (a loud systolic murmur that increases with upright posture or Valsalva and decreases with squatting suggests hypertrophic cardiomyopathy).
	Femoral pulse diminishment suggests aortic coarctation.
Respiratory	Observe for accessory muscle use or prolonged expiration and auscultate for wheezing. Exercise-induced asthma will not produce manifestations on resting examination and requires exercise testing for dx.
Abdominal	Assess for hepatic or splenic enlargement.
GU (males only)	Hernias/varioceles do not usually preclude sports participation, but it may be appropriate to screen for testicular masses..
Musculoskeletal	The "two minute orthopedic exam" is a commonly used systematic screen (refer to the reference below).
	Consider supplemental shoulder, knee, and ankle examinations.
Skin	Evidence of molluscum contagiosum, herpes simplex infection, impetigo, tinea corporis or scabies would temporarily prohibit participation in sports in which direct skin-to-skin competitor contact occurs (i.e., wrestling, martial arts).

Reference: **1. Kurowski K, Chandran S**: The preparticipation athletic evaluation. *Am Fam Physician* 2000;61:2683-98.

3. Conditions that contraindicate sports participation

The following conditions preclude participation: active myocarditis or pericarditis; hypertrophic cardiomyopathy; uncontrolled severe HTN (static resistance exercises are particularly contraindicated); suspected CAD until fully evaluated; long QT interval syndrome; hx of recent concussion and sx of postconcussion syndrome (no contact or collision sports); poorly controlled convulsive disorder (no archery, riflery, swimming, weight lifting, strength training, or sports involving heights); recurrent episodes of burning UEx pain or weakness or episodes of transient quadriplegia until stability of cervical spine can be assured (no contact or collision sports); sickle cell disease (no high exertion, contact, or collision sports); mononucleosis with unresolved splenomegaly; eating disorder where athlete is not compliant with tx or f/u or where there is evidence of diminished performance or potential injury because of eating disorder.

D. Rehabilitation after Hip Fracture

Lifetime risk of hip fx in industrialized countries is 18% for ♀ and 6% for ♂ [1]. Osteoporosis and falls are the primary risk factors. Mortality and morbidity following hip fx are high: 20% are not alive by 1yr post-fx and 33% by 2yrs [2]. Nearly 1 of 3 survivors are in institutionalized care w/in a year after the fx, and as many as 2 of 3 survivors never regain their preoperative activity status [3]. Surgery is usually indicated for most hip fxs, unless medically contraindicated or in nonambulatory pts.

Femoral neck fx - Screw fixations (right) are typical for stable, non-displaced fxs. Ambulation with WBAT and an appropriate assistive device may be started during the first few days post-op. Bipolar endoprostheses (left) may be used for unstable, displaced fxs when satisfactory reduction cannot be achieved and the pt is >65yrs of age or has pre-existing articular pathology (i.e., OA). Pts are usually mobilized quickly and allowed WBAT w/in the first few days post-op. Abduction pillows and short term ROM restrictions (no adduction past midline, no internal rotation) may be ordered to reduce the risk of prosthetic displacement.

Intertrochanteric fx (right) - Sliding hip screw fixation allows for early WBAT for stable fxs (intact posteromedial cortex) and provides dynamic compression of the fx during WB. Intramedullary hip screws are another surgical option. A period of limited WB may be necessary following fixation of unstable fxs. Surgical management for *subtrochanteric fxs* also includes the use of sliding screw fixation and intramedullary nails/rods, although initial WB may be more limited.

Complications seen during rehabilitation and convalescence after hip fx include atelectasis, pneumonia, anemia, fx non-union, avascular necrosis, surgical site infection, component loosening, leg length discrepancy, HO, DVT, constipation, and skin breakdown.

References: **1. Meunier PJ:** Prevention of hip fxs. *Am J Med* 1993;95(suppl):75-8. **2. Emerson S:** 10yr survival after fxs of the proximal end of the femur. *Gerontology* 1988;34:186-91. **3.** Osteoporosis Prevention, Dx, and Therapy. NIH Consensus Statement 2000 March 27-29;17:1-36.

E. Rehabilitation after Joint Replacement

1. Total hip arthroplasty (THA)

Biologically fixed or *"cementless" implants* provide a more durable bioprosthetic interface, but require a longer period of protective WB (i.e., touchdown WB to PWB x ≥2-3mo) to allow for osseous integration into the porous prosthetic surface. *Cement-fixed implants* are cheaper and may offer immediate WBAT. The cement, however, can be prone to deterioration, which may result in component loosening and ultimately require revision.

Pts may be OOB to chair with assist on POD#1. A triangular hip abduction pillow in bed is highly recommended for the first 6-12wks. *Hip precautions* generally continue for up to 12wks post-op to allow for formation of a pseudocapsule and minimize the chance of dislocation. Pts are allowed flexion up to 90°, passive abduction, and gentle (≤30°) internal rotation while extended. There should be no adduction past midline, no external rotation, and no internal rotation while flexed. Active abduction and hyperextension are allowed with a posterior approach (gluteus medius preserved) but avoided after an anterolateral approach (gluteus medius split open). Typical pt instructions are diagrammed below.

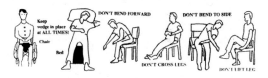

Other key issues include DVT prophylaxis, monitoring for post-op anemia and infection, and pain control. Pts may often complain about perceived leg length discrepancies during the first several months post-op; PT to address muscle imbalances and tight capsules may be helpful. In general, prognosis following THA is excellent, although being younger, male, obese, and highly active may adversely affect outcomes[1].

2. Total knee arthroplasty (TKA)

Cemented fixation may allow immediate WBAT; cementless fixation may require several months of restricted WB for complete stability. Neither addresses the issue of polyethylene liner wear, which may be the key factor in eventual prosthetic failure. Microscopic wear debris can trigger an inflammatory response with ensuing osteolysis and component loosening.

Regaining *knee ROM* (i.e., 0-90° before going home) is an important rehabilitation goal for all TKA pts. Pillows under the knee should be avoided. The use of continuous passive motion (CPM) is controversial. Some have argued that it may decrease length of inpatient rehabilitation stay and improve ROM (by 10°) at 1yr post-op[2], but most studies have *not* demonstrated long term benefits in ROM or functional outcome.

References: 1. 1994 NIH THA Consensus Panel. 2. **Johnson DP**: Beneficial effects of CPM after condylar TKA. *Ann R Coll Surg Engl* 1992;74:412-6. Figure adapted from **DeLisa J**. ed.: *Rehabilitation Medicine: Principles and Practice*, 3rd ed. Lippincott-Raven. 1998.

II. Pain Medicine and the Spine

A. Pain, General Considerations, and Pathophysiology

1.Definitions[1,2] and pain assessment

The International Association for the Study of Pain (IASP) defines pain as an "unpleasant sensory and emotional experience associated with actual or potential tissue damage, or described in terms of such damage"[1]. *Dysesthesia* is "an unpleasant abnormal sensation, whether spontaneous or evoked"[1]. *Paresthesia* is "an abnormal sensation, whether spontaneous or provoked"[1]. (The IASP suggests that the term paresthesia be reserved for abnormal sensations that are *not* unpleasant.) *Hyperalgesia* is "an increased response to a stimulus which is normally painful"[1]. *Allodynia* is "pain due to a stimulus that does not normally provoke pain"[1].

Acute pain is typically localized, self-limited, and due to a readily apparent noxious stimulus. Some practitioners and insurance companies consider *chronic pain* to be pain that lasts >6mos, but it may be better described as pain that exceeds the usual course of an injury or disease. (Chronic pain may last any amount of time, i.e., <6mos or >6mos.) Pts with *chronic pain syndrome* behave in a learned pattern, in order to maintain secondary gains such as narcotic medications and work limitations. They often adopt a new self-image and perceive themselves as "disabled," which may justify their attempts to collect compensation from society[2].

There is no way to directly measure how much pain is experienced. Mental, emotional, social, and behavioral factors will influence pain interpretation. Despite this, several useful clinical tools exist. The 10cm *visual analogue scale* (VAS) has been found to be reproducible, validated, and even more reliable than the numeric verbal rating scale[3]. The *McGill Pain Questionnaire* is useful in the assessment of pts with chronic pain. High scores in the affective domain correlate with greater anxiety and sickness impact, regardless of pain intensity[4]. Multiple studies have shown that unusual distributions on *pain drawings* may correlate with symptom magnification or have psychological significance.

References: 1. **Merskey H.**, ed.: *Classification of Chronic Pain*, 2nd ed., *IASP Task Force on Taxonomy*. IASP Press, 1994. 2. **Walsh NE**: Tx of the pt with chronic pain. In DeLisa J, ed.: *Rehabilitation Medicine: Principles and Practice*, 3rd ed. Lippincott-Raven, 1998. 3. **Ohnhaus EE**: Methodological problems in the measurement of pain: a comparison between the verbal rating scale and the visual analogue scale. *Pain* 1975;1:379-84. 4. **Kremer E**: Pain measurement: construct validity of the affective dimension of the McGill Pain Questionnaire with chronic benign pain pts. *Pain* 1981;11:93-100.

2. Pathophysiology[1]

At right is a simplified model for the production of pain-mediating leukotrienes and prostaglandins after the activation of phospholipases in traumatized or inflamed tissue. These mediators will act directly on primary afferent neurons and will also enhance the nociceptors' response to other inflammatory mediators, e.g., the kinins.

Membrane phospholipids $\xrightarrow{+}$ Trauma, inflammation

$\downarrow$ Phospholipases $\xleftarrow{-}$ Steroids

Arachidonic acid

$\downarrow$ Cyclooxygenase $\longleftarrow$ NSAIDs

Endoperoxides $\xleftarrow{-}$

Leukotrienes

$\downarrow$

Prostaglandins

The nociceptors will, in turn, send ascending signals via *A-δ and C fibers* to the spinal cord. The A-δ fibers synapse primarily in Rexed laminae I and V, while the C fibers primarily synapse in laminae II.

Pain information will next ascend via the spinothalamic and spinoreticular tracts to higher CNS centers. The *neospinothalamic* tract rapidly conveys precise information (e.g., localization) to the posterior ventral thalamus, which then transmits to the postcentral sensory cortex. The *paleospinothalamic* and slow-conducting polysynaptic *spinoreticular* tracts (not pictured) convey poorly localized, dull aching, and burning sensations to the hypothalamus and intralaminar thalamic nuclei, then eventually to the limbic system.

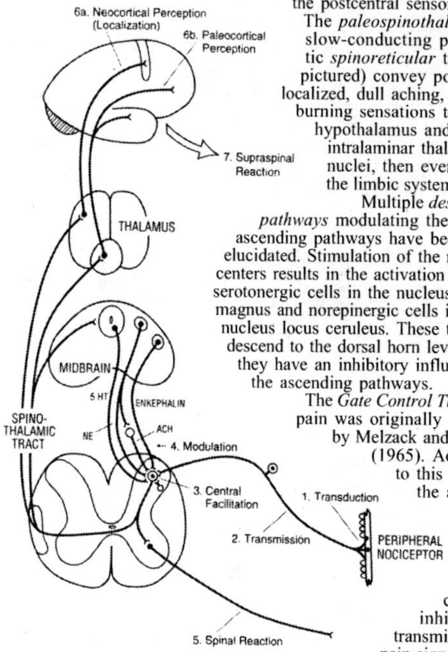

Multiple *descending pathways* modulating the ascending pathways have been elucidated. Stimulation of the midbrain centers results in the activation of serotonergic cells in the nucleus raphe magnus and norepinergic cells in the nucleus locus ceruleus. These tracts descend to the dorsal horn level, where they have an inhibitory influence on the ascending pathways.

The *Gate Control Theory* of pain was originally proposed by Melzack and Wall (1965). According to this theory, the activation of large diameter sensory afferents can inhibit the transmission of pain signals from small-diameter pain fibers through interactions in the substantia gelatinosa of the dorsal horn. This seems to provide a rationale for why rubbing around a painful area or a modality such as TENS might alleviate pain. Anatomic or physiological substantiation of such a model, however, has not been demonstrated.

Figure labels:
- 6a. Neocortical Perception (Localization)
- 6b. Paleocortical Perception
- 7. Supraspinal Reaction
- THALAMUS
- MIDBRAIN
- 5 HT
- ENKEPHALIN
- ACH
- NE
- SPINO-THALAMIC TRACT
- 4. Modulation
- 3. Central Facilitation
- 1. Transduction
- 2. Transmission
- PERIPHERAL NOCICEPTOR
- 5. Spinal Reaction

References: **1.** Walsh NE: Treatment of the patient with chronic pain. In DeLisa J, ed.: *Rehabilitation Medicine: Principles and Practice.* 3rd ed. Lippincott-Raven, 1998. Figure courtesy of Cousins MJ, ed.: *Neural Blockade in Clinical Anesthesia and Management of Pain,* 3rd ed. LWW, 1998.

B. Selected Pain Syndromes

1. Complex regional pain syndrome (CRPS)

In 1994, the IASP replaced the terms "reflex sympathetic dystrophy" and "causalgia" with CRPS type I and type II respectively. The inciting event of CRPS may be traumatic or neurologic (e.g., stroke), and is followed by a period of immobility. Type I is *not* associated with a known nerve injury, while type II *is* associated with a nerve injury. The dx of these syndromes is clinical and is suggested by signs and symptoms such as burning pain, hyperpathia/allodynia, temperature or color changes, edema, or hair/nail growth changes. Characteristic findings on X-ray (patchy osteoporosis) and 3-phase bone scan (see p.120) are also supportive.

CRPS has been classified into stages, but they do not necessarily describe the course of all cases. The *acute (hyperemic) stage* commences at the time of injury or may be delayed for several wks. It may last for a few wks or up to 6mos, and is characterized by constant burning pain, hyperpathia/allodynia, local edema/warmth, and skin changes (e.g., smooth, taut). W/o tx, it may progress to the *dystrophic (ischemic) stage*, which is characterized by a cold, atrophic extremity with ↑ edema, ↑ pain, muscular wasting, patchy osteoporosis, and ↓ function. The *atrophic stage* is characterized by marked trophic changes that are potentially irreversible. There is marked weakness and loss of ROM in the involved joints, which may eventually become ankylosed. Pain, however, may be reduced.

Many different *txs* have been used and advocated, with varying degrees of success. These include PT techniques (e.g., Isotoner gloves, ROM exercises), α-adrenergic blockers (e.g., prazosin, phenoxybenzamine), corticosteroids (e.g., prednisone, 1mg/kg divided into bid dosing for several wks, then tapered), adjuvant pain medications (e.g., TCAs, carbamezepine, gabapentin), IV regional blocks (e.g., Bier blocks), sympathetic blocks (e.g., stellate ganglion for UEx; lumbar sympathetic chain for LEx), sympathetic neurolysis, surgical sympathectomies, and others. Sympathetic blocks in the acute period are generally favored as the most effective tx.

2. Myofascial pain syndrome (MPS)

MPS is a local or regional pain syndrome characterized by exquisitely painful *trigger points* with characteristic patterns of referred pain. In contradistinction to fibromyalgia (FM), fatigue and systemic symptoms are *not* a prominent feature of MPS, and the ♀:♂ ratio is less pronounced (~3:1 for MPS vs. ~10:1 for FM)[1]. MPS trigger points are often accompanied by local, palpable, *taut bands* of muscle that respond with a "twitch response" or "jump sign" when palpated.

Tx options may include direct injection of the trigger points with local anesthetics (e.g., 0.5cc of 1% lidocaine), saline, steroids, botulinum toxin (e.g., up to 100 units BTX-A/trigger point), or even dry needling (e.g., 25-g). Injections should be followed by passive stretch (e.g., x3days). Tx should be w/in the context of a general rehabilitation program emphasizing flexibility. "Myofascial release" and other manual medicine techniques or a stretch-and-spray technique using a vapocoolant spray are also often used.

Reference: **1. Raj P.**, ed.: *Pain Medicine*. Mosby, 1996.

3. Whiplash

Whiplash was originally described to be a syndrome related to cervical acceleration-deceleration injuries (primarily related to hyperextension), but more recently is being used to describe any type of neck injury (usually vehicle-related)[1]. The typical pt is a stationary driver who is struck from behind by another vehicle. Neck muscles may be strained (not macroscopically torn) or torn. Injuries of the cervical spine and/or spinal ligaments (sprains) may also be present. Loss of cervical lordosis due to paraspinal muscle spasms may be noted. Headaches, dizziness, visual disturbances, and medial UEx paresthesiae (ulnar distribution) are common associated findings. Often the pt may not be aware of injury at the time of the accident and only become symptomatic hours afterwards. Segmental dysfunction and facet-mediated pain are common.

Tx involves local heat, NSAIDs, and muscle relaxants. The Quebec Task Force suggests restricting the use of soft collars to a minimum, advising that prolonged use is detrimental[2]. Driving should be avoided. Generally, in the absence of major anatomic injury, 2wks of conservative tx should yield significant improvement[3]. If not, 2 more wks of the same regimen with the possible addition of light home cervical traction can be considered[3]. If h/a is persistent at 4wks post-injury, a cranial CT can be considered; if arm/shoulder pain is persistent at 4wks, a spinal MRI can be considered[3].

References: 1. **Nachemson A**, ed.: *Neck and Back Pain: The Scientific Evidence of Causes, Dx, and Tx.* LWW, 2000. 2. Spitzer WO: Scientific monograph of the Quebec Task Force on whiplash-associated disorders: redefining "whiplash" and its management. *Spine* 1995;20(8Suppl):1S-73S. 3. **Borenstein DG**: *Neck Pain: Medical Dx and Comprehensive Management.* WB Saunders, 1996. Figure courtesy of **Fu F, Stone D**: *Sports Injuries: Mechanisms, Prevention & Tx.* Williams & Wilkins, 1994.

4. Low back pain (LBP)

Introduction and epidemiology of LBP - Most surveys define LBP as pain occurring between the costal margins and gluteal folds and ask about pain lasting >24hrs[1]. International surveys of LBP report a point prevalence of 15-30% and a lifetime prevalence of 60-70%[1]. In a telephone survey of ~4000 U.S. adults, Carey found that the prevalence of functionally limiting LBP was 8.5% among adults <60y/o and 5% >60y/o[2]. Just over 1% of Americans are permanently disabled by LBP, and another 1% are temporarily disabled by LBP at any given time[1].

Most pts, however, will *not* have anatomically defined lesions. After 1 month of symptoms, only ~15% of pts will have a definable disease or injury[1]. This proportion is even lower in the first few days post-injury[1]. In a study of primary care pts, Deyo found that at ~4wks, 4-5% had disk herniation, 4-5% had symptoms of spinal stenosis, 4% had a compression fx, and 1% had a primary metastatic tumor or osteomyelitis[3]. <1% had a visceral disease, aortic aneurysm, or a renal or gynecological disorder[3].

References: 1. **Nachemson A**, ed.: *Neck and Back Pain: The Scientific Evidence of Causes, Dx, and Tx.* LWW, 2000. 2. Carey TS: Acute, severe LBP: a population-based study of prevalence and care-seeking. *Spine* 1996;21:339-44. 3. **Deyo RA**: What can the H&P tell us about LBP? *JAMA* 1992;268:760-5.

Key elements in the H&P of a LBP pt[1,2,3]

A clear description of the onset, character, radiation, alleviating/aggravating factors, and previous tx of the pain should be obtained. Mechanical LBP is "achy" and improves with rest. Discogenic pain can be burning and constant. Pain radiating below the knee is more likely to represent a true radiculopathy than pain radiating only to the posterior thigh. Numbness or weakness in the legs further increases the likelihood of neurologic involvement. Bladder dysfunction (especially retention) and saddle anesthesia suggest possible cauda equina involvement. Failure of bed rest to relieve pain is a sensitive but nonspecific finding for malignancy.

Other historical elements can raise or lower the probability of an underlying systemic disease. The most useful items include age, h/o cancer, duration of pain, unexplained weight loss, and responsiveness to previous therapy. IVDA or UTI raise the suspicion of spinal infection. A psychosocial hx, including a hx of substance abuse, disability compensation, or previous failed txs, can help to estimate prognosis and plan therapy.

The *physical exam* should include observation of posture and gait. On inspection, ↓ lumbar lordosis may be indicative of disc or vertebral body collapse. ↑ lordosis may be seen with high grade spondylolisthesis or in the obese. A rapid neurologic screen for uncomplicated pts can emphasize ADF and EHL strength, ankle DTRs, and pinprick exam of the medial (L4), dorsal (L5), and lateral (S1) aspects of the foot. Muscle weakness is generally considered a more reliable indicator of nerve compression than other components of the exam. Diminished reflexes may be noted with LMN lesions (e.g., lumbar stenosis). In pts with sciatica or possible neurogenic claudication, b/l straight leg raising (SLR) should be assessed, preferably with a goniometer. The test is positive if pain radiates below the knee. Stretch of the sciatic nerve is greatest between ~35-70° of hip flexion on the SLR. A +SLR at >70° is more likely to be due to joint pain.

Examination of the soft tissues may reveal myofascial trigger points, which may be the etiology or a component of the pt's LBP syndrome. Intense vertebral tenderness is a sensitive but nonspecific finding for infection.

Waddell's signs of non-organic LBP are commonly used to assess pain behaviors, and have demonstrated reliability and validity in the clinical setting. If ≥3 of the 5 signs below are positive, then a non-organic basis for the physical complaints is likely and the exam is invalidated. Waddell's signs are more sensitive in chronic back pain than in acute back pain.

Waddell's signs:
a. *Regionalization* - regional weakness/sensory loss.
b. *Overreaction* - exaggerated pain response to non-painful stimulus.
c. *Simulation* - e.g., LBP on axial loading or sham rotation of the spine.
d. *Distraction* - inconsistent findings during distraction.
e. *Tenderness* - non-anatomic or superficial.

References: 1. **Nachemson A.**, ed.: *Neck and Back Pain: The Scientific Evidence of Causes, Dx, and Tx.* LWW, 2000. 2. **Deyo RA**: Cancer as the cause of back pain frequency, clinical presentation, and diagnostic strategies. *J Gen Int Med* 1988;3:230-8. 3. **Deyo RA**: What can the H&P tell us about LBP? *JAMA* 1992;268:760-5.

Laboratory tests and imaging of the LBP pt

Some potentially useful, but nonspecific, lab tests include alkaline phosphatase (Paget's disease, osteomalacia), amylase (pancreatitis), ESR (cancer, polymyalgia rheumatica), pregnancy test (ectopic pregnancy), RF/ANA (rheumatic disease), and urinalysis (prostatitis, renal stones).

Plain *x-rays* for suspected spondylolisthesis should be done with the pt standing, as some cases of spondylolisthesis may reduce in the supine position. Plain films may also show arthritic changes, diffuse idiopathic skeletal hyperostosis, or spondylolisthesis. A *CT* or *MRI* can be considered for back pain failing conservative management if a structural lesion is suspected (e.g., herniated disk), although there is no evidence that either modality has improved the treatment of common back syndromes[1]. For back pain with adverse features, such as severe or progressive neurologic deficit, urgent specialist referral and MRI should be considered.

Conservative tx of the LBP pt

Acute LBP[1] - There is strong evidence in the literature that *NSAIDs* at regular intervals provide effective pain relief in simple acute LBP, but do not affect return to work, natural history, or chronicity of pain. There is also strong evidence that the different types of NSAIDs are equally effective. Five high quality RCTs demonstrated better improvement in pain intensity using *muscle relaxants* versus placebo. Drowsiness and dependency issues, however, can be significant, even with short-term use. Only limited evidence regarding *oral steroids* is available, and it suggests that oral steroids are probably *not* effective for acute LBP.

There is moderate evidence that *manipulation* is more effective than placebo for short-term relief of acute LBP. It is *not* clear, however, if it is *more* effective than PT approaches (e.g., massage, heat modalities, exercises) or analgesics. Nonetheless, the risks of manipulation are low in trained practitioners' hands. Pts with severe or progressive neurologic deficits, however, should *not* undergo manipulation.

A metaanalysis of 10 RCTs revealed that *bed rest* is *not* effective for treating acute LBP. Additionally, there are complications to immobilization, including muscle wasting and bone mineral loss.

The literature regarding numerous other txs, such as *specific back exercises*, *"back schools,"* *traction*, *corsets*, and *TENS* is conflicting. Moreover, many of these studies have methodological limitations precluding the development of clear clinical guidelines. Generally, isometric flexion exercises for chronic LBP, stretching, and the use of early, aggressive work-hardening programs are supported, although the data are not high-quality.

Chronic LBP[1] - The literature strongly supports manual therapy, exercise therapy, multidisciplinary pain tx programs, and spa therapy, especially for short-term benefits. NSAIDs may help some pts with chronic LBP return to usual activities; but convincing evidence supporting TENS, EMG biofeedback, orthoses, or acupuncture for the same purpose has yet to be reported. No evidence supports any form of long-term maintenance tx.

References: **1. Nachemson A**, ed.: *Neck and Back Pain: The Scientific Evidence of Causes, Dx, and Tx.* LWW, 2000.

Selected LBP syndromes[1,2]

Internal disk disruption (IDD) - The intervertebral disk is a poorly vascularized tissue that tends not to heal well. Microtrauma and annular tears may result in the release of inflammatory mediators such as phospholipase A_2 that may eventually lead to the activation of local pain fibers, e.g., in the outer third of the disk annulus, the posterior longitudinal ligament, vertebral body, dural sac, and epidural vascular structures.

Risks for IDD include repetitive twisting and prolonged sitting. Onset is typically insidious. Pain can be exacerbated by lifting, coughing, sitting, standing, or transitional movements (e.g., arising from a chair).

Dx is by discography or CT-discography. Tx is controversial, with some proponents for aggressive conservative care, and other proponents for surgical fusion. An epidural steroid injection may be helpful. Recently, *intradiscal electrothermy* (IDET) has also been advocated for the tx of IDD. Ideally, the pain source (annulus fibrosis) should be confirmed with a discogram first. The thermal energy applied to the collagen of the disk may cause the formation of a fibrotic scar and desensitize the annulus to pain. Additionally, any concomitant nucleus pulposus bulges may be reduced. The best outcomes are said to follow single disk IDET.

Lumbar radiculopathy - Radiculopathies may be due to herniated disks, bony stenosis, mass lesions, or other causes. The majority of clinically significant lumbar disk herniations occur at L4-5 and L5-S1, causing L5 and S1 radiculopathies respectively.

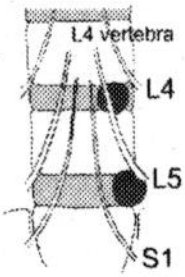

Useful symptoms and signs in the dx of lumbar radiculopathy with good interrater reliability and positive predictive value include crossed straight leg raising (SLR) (the best test), a positive SLR at <60° reproducing leg pain, pain at night, severe radicular pain, unilateral leg pain worse than back pain, and loss of lordosis. (A crossed SLR test is positive when there is pain in the symptomatic [non-raised] leg when the asymptomatic leg is raised.)

Fig.1: A posterolateral L4-5 disk herniation spares the L4 root, but encroaches on the L5 root. A very far lateral L5-S1 hernia can compress the L5 root.

Although commonly performed in the clinical setting, CT or MRI is probably most useful when surgery is being considered or if a malignancy is suspected. EDx studies can help localize a lesion and should be considered particularly if imaging studies and clinical findings conflict.

Tx - There is limited evidence that *epidural steroids* are more effective than placebo or bed rest for acute LBP with radicular symptoms. There is no evidence that they are helpful in acute LBP w/o radicular symptoms. Caudal epidurals are most effective for S1 nerve root lesions. Incorrect needle placements have been noted ~25-40% of the time epidurals are attempted w/o fluoroscopic guidance. Complications include vascular injections, direct trauma to the nerve, abscesses, hematomas, urinary retention, h/a, and spinal block. *Surgical interventions* should be reserved for central disk herniations with bowel or bladder dysfunction and LEx weakness or for pts who continue to have pain and dysfunction despite an adequate trial of conservative tx.

Lumbar spinal stenosis - Stenosis can be noted in various portions of the spinal canal, including the lateral recesses or central canal. Criteria for clinically significant stenosis vary, e.g., AP diameters of <7mm or <10mm on CT or MRI, cross-sectional areas <70mm^2 on CT myelogram.

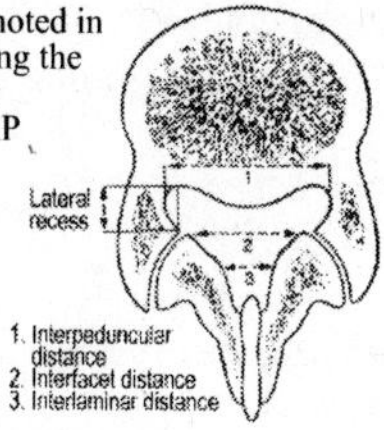

1. Interpeduncular distance
2. Interfacet distance
3. Interlaminar distance

Fig.2

The most common historical feature noted with lumbar central canal stenosis is a reduced walking distance. The symptoms are usually of gradual onset and consistent with neurogenic claudication (e.g., pain after standing or walking, worse when walking downhill, worse with lumbar extension, or relieved with flexion). Pain radiating to the buttocks and b/l LEx is common. On exam, there may be ↓ reflexes. SLR tests are typically negative.

Tx is aggressive conservative care, possibly with lumbar bracing in a mildly flexed position. Aquatic therapy may help alleviate spinal loading and improve symptoms. Surgical decompression with or w/o fusion should be considered in pts with persistent or progressive symptoms or neurologic deficits.

Lumbar zygapophyseal (facet) arthropathy - Facet arthropathy may be due to traumatic or degenerative processes. Pts typically complain of generalized LBP, sometimes with radiation to the buttocks or posterior thigh but not below the knee. Pain may be exacerbated with spinal extension, lateral bending, and rotation towards affected side; pain is relieved by lumbar flexion. The H&P and plain films, however, have *not* been shown to accurately correlate with facet joint pain. Fluoroscopically-guided, contrast-enhanced intraarticular or medial branch local anesthetic blocks are diagnostic for painful facets. A medial branch block that temporarily decreases pain may be followed by a radiofrequency ablation of the same nerves, which should provide more long-lasting relief.

Spondylolysis/spondylolisthesis - Spondylolysis is a defect of the pars interarticularis and may be congenital or due to repetitive traumatic stress. L5 and, to a lesser degree, L4 are commonly involved. Spondylolisthesis is a subluxation of one vertebra on another and is seen most commonly at the lumbosacral junction. Causes include spondylolysis, degenerative changes, Paget's disease, and bony dysplasia.

Heat, massage, and stretching of the hip flexors, hamstrings, and Achilles tendons are the mainstays of tx for spondylolysis with ≤ grade II spondylolisthesis. Back orthoses and abdominal strengthening exercises may help reduce pain. Lumbar flexion or isometric exercises are thought to be more effective for improving pain and function than extension exercises. *Laminectomy and surgical fusion* to secure the unstable segment and reduce the irritation on compressed nerves may be required for grade III or IV spondylolisthesis or for the pt with neurologic symptoms.

References: **1. Nachemson A**, ed.: *Neck and Back Pain: The Scientific Evidence of Causes, Dx, and Tx*. LWW, 2000. **2. Frontera WR**, ed.: *Essentials of PM&R*. Hanley & Belfus, 2002. **Fig.2** courtesy of **Cox JM**, ed.: *Low Back Pain: Mechanism, Dx, and Tx*. LWW, 1999.

III. MODALITIES

A. Essential Points of a Modalities Rx

1. Diagnosis
2. Impairments/disabilities
3. Precautions
4. Modality
5. Area to be treated
6. Intensity/settings/temp range
7. Frequency of treatment
8. Duration of treatment
9. Goals/objectives of treatment
10. Date of re-evaluation

B. Selected Modalities

Heat - The therapeutic temperature range is 40-45°C. Heat should be maintained for 5-30mins. Superficial heat is considered to be 1-2cm; deep heat: 3.5-8cm.

Conduction is transfer of heat by contact, e.g., paraffin baths and hot packs (e.g., Hydrocollator packs). Although paraffin bath temperatures are ~52-54°C, poor heat conductivity allows tolerance. *Convection* involves the flow of heat, e.g., fluidotherapy, whirlpool, moist air. Examples of *conversion* (where non-thermal energy converts to heat) include infrared, ultrasound (US), shortwave diathermy (SWD) and microwave diathermy (MWD). Infrared has a 2cm depth penetration. US penetrates 3.5-8cm; the greatest heating is at the bone-tissue interface. US parameters include a frequency of 0.8-1.1 MHz; intensity of 0.5-4 W/cm^2; treatment area of ~100cm^2; and duration of 5-8min. SWD penetrates 4-5 cm; fat is heated more than muscle; the most commonly used frequency is 27.12MHz. MWD is rarely used. Penetration is not as deep as SWD; the 915MHz frequency penetrates deeper than 2450MHz.

Contraindications to heat therapy include acute hemorrhage or bleeding dyscrasia, inflammation, malignancy, insensate skin, inability to respond to pain, atrophic skin, and ischemia. Contraindications for *US* also include treatment over fluid-filled cavities (e.g., eyes, uterus), or near a pace-maker, laminectomy site, or joint prostheses. *SWD* should not be used for children (immature epiphyses) and persons with metallic implants, contact lenses, or menstruating/pregnant uteri. *MWD* should not be used over the eyes due to the risk of developing cataracts.

Cryotherapy - Cold, unlike heat, is limited to superficial applications only. The physiological effects of cold include hemodynamic vasoconstriction and slowing of NCV (via conduction block, i.e., C and A-δ fibers). Group Ia firing rates are likewise decreased, reducing the muscle stretch reflex (and thereby reducing spasticity). Cold is *contraindicated* in the setting of ischemia, insensate skin, severe HTN, or cold sensitivity syndromes (i.e., Raynaud's syndrome, cryoglobinemia, and cold allergy).

Traction

Cervical traction - About 25-30lbs of force is recommended for cervical traction (about 10 of those pounds is used to overcome the effects of gravity, i.e., the weight of the head). The intervertebral space is greatest at 30° of flexion; extension is not recommended due to vertebrobasilar insufficiency.

Lumbar traction - A force of 26% of the body weight is needed to overcome the effects of friction when lying supine with the hips and knees flexed[1]. An additional 25% of body weight is needed to achieve vertebral separation. A split lumbar traction table can essentially eliminate the frictional component. Although often prescribed for back pain (e.g., herniated disks, radiculopathy), the efficacy of this modality is not clear.

General *contraindications* for spinal traction include ligamentous instability, osteomyelitis, discitis, bone malignancy, spinal cord tumor, severe osteoporosis, and untreated HTN. Contraindications specific to *C-spine* traction include vertebrobasilar artery insufficiency, RA, midline herniated disk, and acute torticollis. Contraindications specific to *L-spine* traction include restrictive lung disease, pregnancy, active peptic ulcers, aortic aneurysm, gross hemorrhoids, and cauda equina syndrome.

Transcutaneous electrical nerve stimulation (TENS) - Several theories explaining the mechanism of action of TENS exist. In the "gate theory" introduced by Melzack and Wall[2], stimulation of large myelinated fibers (A-β and A-γ) stimulates interneurons in the substantia gelatinosa, which in turn exert an inhibitory influence on Lamina V, where the small unmyelinated A-δ and C pain fibers synapse with spinal neurons.

"*Conventional*" or high-frequency (50-100Hz) TENS uses barely perceptible, low amplitude, short duration signals. Periodic adjustments to the pulse width and frequency may be necessary, due to accommodations to the settings. "*Acupuncture-like*" TENS uses larger amplitude, low-frequency (1-4Hz) signals that may be uncomfortable. β-endorphin release may play a role in the analgesic effects. *Contraindications* to TENS include use near pacemakers (controversial), gravid uteri, and carotid sinuses.

Massage - Classic Western techniques include *effleurage* (stroking), *petrissage* (kneading), *tapotment* (percussion), and *Swedish* (tapotment + petrissage + deep tissue massage). *Deep friction massage* is used to break up adhesions in chronic muscle injuries. *Myofascial release* attempts to release soft tissue entrapped in tight fascia through the prolonged application of light pressure in specific directions. *Eastern techniques* include acupressure and Shiatsu massage.

Absolute contraindications to massage include malignancy, DVT, atherosclerotic plaques, and infected tissues. *Relative contraindications* include incompletely healed scar tissue, anticoagulation, calcified soft tissues, and skin grafts.

Phonophoresis - Topical medications (e.g., steroids, anesthetics) are mixed with an acoustic coupling medium, which are then driven into the tissue by US. Common uses include OA, bursitis, capsulitis, tendonitis, strains, contractures, scar tissue, and neuromas.

Iontophoresis - Electrical currents are used to drive medications across biological membranes into the symptomatic areas, while theoretically avoiding the systemic side effects of the medications.

References: **1. Judovich BD**: Lumbar traction therapy: elimination of physical factors that prevent lumbar stretch. *JAMA* 1955;159:549-50. **2. Melzack R, Wall PD**: Pain mechanisms: a new theory. *Science* 1965;150:971-9.

IV. GAIT AND GAIT AIDS
A. Gait Cycle

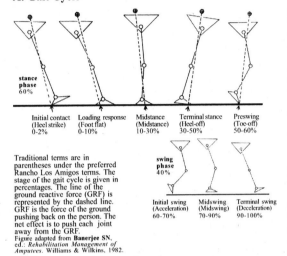

| Initial contact (Heel strike) 0-2% | Loading response (Foot flat) 0-10% | Midstance (Midstance) 10-30% | Terminal stance (Heel-off) 30-50% | Preswing (Toe-off) 50-60% |

stance phase 60%

Traditional terms are in parentheses under the preferred Rancho Los Amigos terms. The stage of the gait cycle is given in percentages. The line of the ground reactive force (GRF) is represented by the dashed line. GRF is the force of the ground pushing back on the person. The net effect is to push each joint away from the GRF.

Figure adapted from **Banerjee SN**, ed.: *Rehabilitation Management of Amputees.* Williams & Wilkins, 1982.

swing phase 40%

| Initial swing (Acceleration) 60-70% | Midswing (Midswing) 70-90% | Terminal swing (Deceleration) 90-100% |

B. The Six Determinants of Gait[1]

Saunders et al. began by assuming that gait is most efficient when vertical and lateral excursions of the body's center of gravity (COG) are minimized. They identified 6 naturally occurring "determinants" in normal gait that reduced these excursions and suggested that pathological gait could be identified when these determinants were compromised.

1. Pelvic rotation in the horizontal plane - The pelvis rotates 4° to each side, which occurs maximally during double support, elevating the nadir of the COG pathway curve about 3/8".

2. Pelvic tilt in the frontal plane - The pelvis drops 5° on the side of the swinging leg, shaving 3/16" from the apex of the COG pathway curve.

3. Knee flexion - KF lowers the COG 7/16" during midstance.

4, 5. Knee and ankle motion - These two determinants smoothen the pathway of the COG at the nadir, making it more sinusoidal.

6. Lateral pelvic displacement - Normal valgus at the knee decreases lateral sway, reducing total horizontal excursion from about 6" to <2".

Reference: **1. Saunders JB, Inman VT, Eberhart HD**: The major determinants in normal and pathological gait. *JBJS (Am)* 1953;35:543-58.

C. Muscle Activity during Nondisabled Gait

Ankle dorsiflexors - These muscles (primarily the tibialis anterior, but also the extensor digitorum longus and extensor hallucis longus) eccentrically contract to smoothly lower the foot from heel strike to foot flat. They also concentrically contract during swing phase to dorsiflex the ankle and effectively shorten the swinging limb in order to clear the ground.

Ankle plantarflexors - The triceps surae act eccentrically during midstance to control ankle dorsiflexion caused by the body's forward momentum. At push off, they act concentrically to lift the heel and toes off the ground.

Hip abductors - The gluteus medius and minimus contract eccentrically during stance phase to limit pelvic tilt of the swing phase leg.

Hip flexors - The hip flexors (primarily the iliopsoas) contract eccentrically after midstance phase to slow truncal extension caused by the GRF passing behind the hip. The tensor fasciae latae, pectineus, sartorius, and iliopsoas contract concentrically to flex the hip and shorten the limb for effective ground clearance during swing phase.

Hip extensors - The gluteus maximus and hamstrings start to eccentrically contract just before heel strike to maintain hip stability and slow down the forward momentum of the trunk, since the GRF is anterior to hip at this stage. They become essentially inactive after foot flat, once the GRF passes posterior to the hip. The hamstrings may weakly contract during swing phase to flex the knee for ground clearance.

Knee extensors - The quadriceps act primarily to absorb shock during heel strike and keep the knee stable by eccentric contraction. They are also active just before toe-off to help initiate the forward swing of the limb.

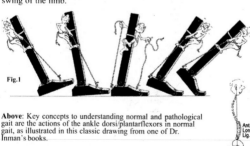

Fig.1

Above: Key concepts to understanding normal and pathological gait are the actions of the ankle dorsi/plantarflexors in normal gait, as illustrated in this classic drawing from one of Dr. Inman's books.

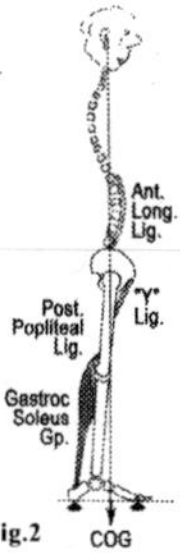

Right: The gastroc-soleus complex (primarily the soleus) is the only muscle normally active during quiet standing. Ligaments and bony articulations maintain the stability of the other joints. The center of gravity (COG) is located ~2" anterior to S2.

Ant.
Long.
Lig.

Post.
Popliteal
Lig.

"Y"
Lig.

Gastroc
Soleus
Gp.

Fig.2   COG

Fig.1 courtesy of **Inman V**: *Human Walking*. Williams & Wilkins, 1981. **Fig.2** courtesy of **Cailliet R**: *Low Back Pain Syndromes*, 5th ed. FA Davis, 1995.

D. Gait Deviations and Prescriptions

Antalgic gait - To reduce pain, there is avoidance of weight bearing on the affected limb. The examiner may note a decrease in the stance phase, a reduced step length on the unaffected side, and a prolonged period of double support.

Gastrocnemius gait - Weak plantarflexors during terminal stance and toe-off prevent adequate heel lift. To limit the drop in the center of gravity that occurs without heel lift during terminal stance, the step length of the contralateral leg is shortened. *Tx* - An AFO with a long sole shank simulates plantar flexion during terminal stance.

Gluteus medius-minimus (Trendelenburg) gait

- In an uncompensated Trendelenburg gait, there is contralateral pelvic drop secondary to the inability of the hip abductors to stabilize the pelvis during stance. A lateral lurch over the affected side is a compensatory maneuver to reduce the stress on the weak muscles. *Tx* - A cane used in the contralateral hand widens the base of support and decreases the hip abductor strength needed to keep the pelvis level. In b/l abductor weakness, b/l canes with a four-point gait may be used.

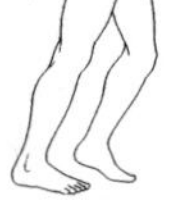

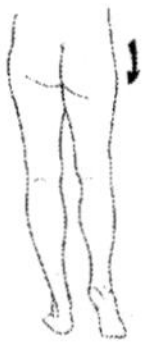

Fig.1
uncompensated
Trendelenberg

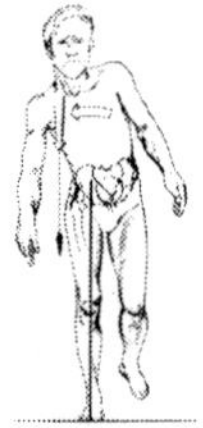

Fig.2
compensated
Trendelenberg

⇨**Gluteus maximus (extensor lurch) gait** - This may be seen following injury to the inferior gluteal nerve or a subtrochanteric hip fx. Weakened hip extensors are unable to decelerate the forward momentum of the body (hip flexion moment) at heel strike. To compensate, the subject adopts a prominent posterior lean to keep the body's center of gravity behind the hip. *Tx* - Two crutches or canes are used for a three-point gait.

Fig.3

Hemiplegic gait - Pts with extensor synergies will typically ambulate independently. The extensor tone effectively makes the plegic limb longer than the nonplegic side. This may be compensated by a circumducted gait to allow toe clearance. Despite the circumduction, there is a decreased step length and swing phase on the plegic side. Gait speed will be reduced in order to maintain an acceptable rate of energy expenditure. *Tx* - A solid AFO to decrease effective limb length may be helpful. A small degree of plantarflexion, however, should be maintained to promote knee stability.

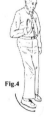

Fig.4

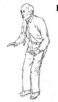

Parkinsonian gait - The classic triad of Parkinson's disease is tremor, bradykinesia, and instability, with at least the last two affecting gait. While standing, the knees, trunk, and neck are typically flexed and the body appears stiff. When ambulation is engaged, there is a characteristic shuffling gait with short quickening steps, as if the patient were racing after the center of gravity (festination). Turns are made "en bloc." Decreased armswing further compromises balance. *Tx* - Heel lifts and assistive devices may help reduce the tendency to fall backwards. Walkers with added weight may provide additional stability. Physical therapy to address postural issues can be helpful.

Fig.5

Quadriceps (back knee) gait - With weakness or inhibition of the quadriceps (e.g., distal femoral fx), the subject will adopt measures to prevent buckling of the knee. One compensation is the use of the hands (**Fig.6**) to force the knee into extension. Also, pts may lurch their trunks forward at initial contact and strongly contract their ankle plantarflexors to bring the center of gravity in front of the knee and force it into extension. Another compensatory technique might be to externally rotate the leg at initial contact and early stance to prevent it from buckling. *Tx* - A knee brace may be used to provide knee stability at heel strike.

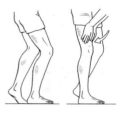

Fig.6

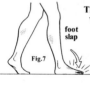

foot slap

Fig.7

Tibialis anterior gait - Pretibial muscle weakness that is at least antigravity (≥3/5 grade) may cause *foot slap* after heel strike. If the muscles are <3/5, foot slap is generally *not* heard because a *steppage gait* is more likely. The hip and knee are hyperflexed in a steppage gait to clear the foot during swing phase, which may otherwise drag. The affected limb may alternatively be circumducted during swing phase. *Tx* - A standard AFO is often used both to prevent foot slap and to allow clearance of the foot during swing phase. Note that ankle plantarflexion stabilizes the knee. Thus, a standard AFO (with plantar flexion stop) may destabilize the knee. An alternative is a posterior spring, which allows plantarflexion and assists in dorsiflexion.

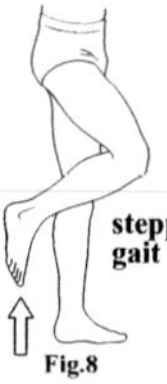

steppage gait

Fig.8

Figs.1,4,5 courtesy of **Magee D**: *Orthopedic Physical Assessment*, 3rd ed. WB Saunders, 1997.

E. Gait Aids[1,2]

1. Cane basics

a. In general, a cane should be held in the hand opposite to the lower limb with neuromuscular weakness or joint pathology, and is advanced with the affected limb together in a *three-point gait* pattern. Stairs are usually ascended with the stronger lower limb first, then the cane and affected limb. The affected lower limb and cane proceed down first during stair descent. ("Up with the good, down with the bad.") In practice, however, there are no hard and fast rules.

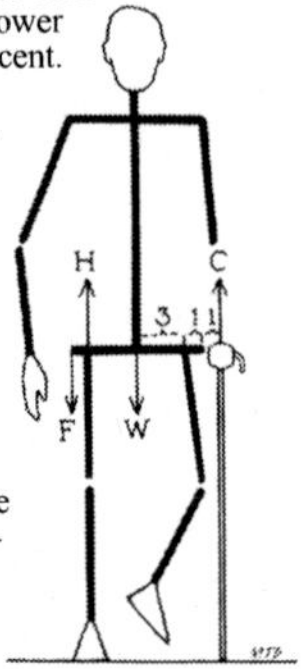

b. Cane length should be from the bottom of the shoe's heel to the upper border of the *greater trochanter* with the pt standing. The shoulders should be level and the arm holding the cane should be *flexed ~20-30° at the elbow*, to provide proper push-off. A cane can unload up to 20% of body weight off the affected lower limb, depending on cane design and the pt's level of training.

c. The basis for holding a cane on the opposite side of hip joint pathology is elegantly described elsewhere[1]. In essence, the cane provides a rotatory moment (**C**, on picture to the right) that counteracts the weight of the body (**W**) and reduces the force of the gluteus medius (**F**) necessary to maintain equilibrium at the hip fulcrum (**H**) when the affected lower limb is in single support stance phase.

Fig.1

2. Crutch basics

a. Crutches have 2 points of contact with the body and are thus more stable than canes. Shoulder depressors (latissimus dorsi and pectoralis major) are important muscles in ambulation with crutches. Other important muscles to strengthen in preparation for crutch use include the triceps brachii, biceps brachii, quadriceps, hip extensors and hip abductors.

b. *Axillary crutch* length is 1-2" plus the distance from the anterior axillary fold to a point on the ground 6" lateral to the bottom of the heel while standing. The handpiece is placed with the *elbow flexed 30°*, the wrist in extension, and the fingers forming a fist. The pt should be able to raise the body 1-2" by complete elbow extension. Use of heavy padding on the axillary area of the crutch, although a popular practice, should be discouraged. This encourages the habit of resting the body on the crutches, which increases the risk of *compressive radial neuropathies*. When used properly, b/l crutches can provide total WB relief to a lower limb.

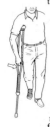

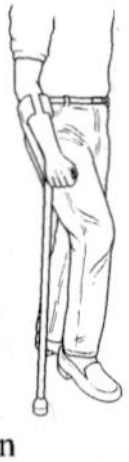

c. *Forearm crutches* (Lofstrand) are indicated if pressure in the axilla is contraindicated, e.g., open wound, compression neuropathy. They provide less trunk support than axillary crutches. A single forearm crutch can relieve up to 40-50% of body weight off a lower limb. B/l forearm crutches can provide total WB relief to a lower limb.

d. *Crutch gaits*

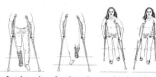

2-point gait   **3-point gait**   **4-point gait**

The crutches and involved limb serve as 1
point, while the uninvolved limb is the 2nd
point in the *2-point (or "hop-to") gait*. In
the *3-point gait* (i.e., the involved limb is
PWB), the crutches (1 point) and each limb
(points 2 and 3) are advanced separately with
any 2 of the 3 points maintaining contact with

the ground at all times. In the *4-point gait* above, point 3 is the
involved leg. Each point is advanced separately. Efficiency is
forsaken for increased stability or balance. When negotiating stairs
w/o a banister, one method might be: stronger limb→weaker limb→
crutch→crutch for ascent; crutch→crutch→weaker limb→stronger
limb for descent. A rail or banister, if present, replaces one of the
crutches in the above method.

3. Walker basics

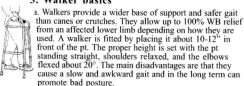

a. Walkers provide a wider base of support and safer gait
than canes or crutches. They allow up to 100% WB relief
from an affected lower limb depending on how they are
used. A walker is fitted by placing it about 10-12" in
front of the pt. The proper height is set with the pt
standing straight, shoulders relaxed, and the elbows
flexed about 20°. The main disadvantages are that they
cause a slow and awkward gait and in the long term can
promote bad posture.

b. *Rolling walkers* are indicated for pts who lack the
coordination or strength in the upper limbs to lift and advance a
standard walker and are preferred in the rehab of total joint
replacement b/c of the smoother gait.

c. A *hemiwalker* is used by a hemiplegic. It is wide-based, provides
more lateral support than a quad-cane, and is advanced by the nonplegic side.

d. *Platform walkers* (right) are used in a variety of
situations including distal UEx joint deformities, grip
weakness, and flexion contractures of the elbow. They
allow weight bearing at the elbow, bypassing the hand,
wrist and part of the forearm, and are useful for patients
with multiple fractures that may preclude use of a non-
platform device.   **Fig.2**

References: **1. Deathe AB**: The biomechanics of canes, crutches, and walkers. *Crit Rev Phys Med Rehab* 1993;5:15-29. **2. Blount WP**: Don't throw away the cane. *JBJS (Am)* 1956;38:695-8. **3. Kottke F.**, ed.: *Krusen's Handbook of PM&R*, 4th ed. WB Saunders, 1990. **Fig.1** courtesy of **Kottke F.**, ed.: *Krusen's Handbook of PM&R*, 4th ed. WB Saunders, 1990. **Fig.2** courtesy of **Redford J.**, ed.: *Orthotics Etcetera*, 3rd ed. Williams & Wilkins, 1986.

V. AMPUTATION/PROSTHETICS

A. Epidemiology[1], Etiology[1], Levels of Amputation

Incidence is ~70,000 major amputations/yr in the U.S. ~65% of all amputations are due to PVD, often due to DM. Nearly half of all diabetic amputees will lose the other leg w/in 5yrs. **Traumatic amputations** (~25%) are more commonly seen in young adults; the right side is more often affected in work-related UEx amputations. **Malignancy** is responsible for ~5% of amputations and is seen more commonly in 10-20 year olds. **Congenital limb deficiency** comprises ~5% of all amputations.

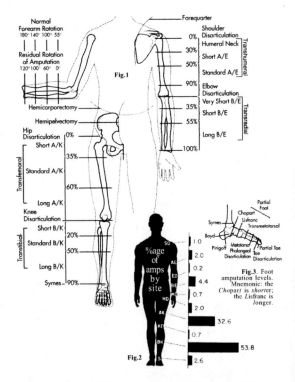

Fig.1

Fig.2

Fig.3. Foot amputation levels. Mnemonic: the *Chopart* is *shorter*; the *Lisfranc* is *longer*.

References: 1. **Eftekhari N**: Amputation rehabilitation. In **O'Young BJ**, ed.: *PMR Secrets*, 2nd ed. Hanley & Belfus, 2002. **Figs.1,3** courtesy of **Tan J**: *Practical Manual of PM&R*. Mosby, 1998. **Fig.2** courtesy of **Muilenberg AL**: *A Manual for Above-Knee Amputees*, 4th ed. The Academy of Orthotists and Prosthetists, 1994.

Preferred mature residual limb length and shape

Transhumeral - Cylindrical appendage with retention of the deltoid tuberosity. Generally, the longer the better (up to 90% of normal length).

Transradial - Ideal shape follows the contours of the natural limb. Longer appendages provide better lever arms, more pronation/supination, and are optimal for body-powered prostheses and heavy labor. Retention of the brachioradialis improves elbow flexion. Medium length limbs are optimal for externally-powered prostheses.

Transfemoral - Ideal shape is conical. Longer residual limbs improve seating balance and tolerance. For shorter limbs, maintaining the greater trochanter and its attachment to the hip abductors is key.

Transtibial - Ideal shape and length is a cylindrical appendage about one-third the original tibial length, with retention of the patellar tendon attachment to the tibial tuberosity. The fibula should be shorter than the tibia. In vascular disease, longer limbs may not have adequate circulatory supply.

B. Basic LEx Post-Amputation Preprosthetic Care[1]

1. Residual limb shaping - If figure-of-8 *elastic wrapping*, e.g., ACE bandaging, is to be used (shown for a transtibial amputation below), it should begin immediately after surgery and should ideally be rewrapped qid. Circumferential wraps can trap edema distally. Once the scar has healed, *elastic shrinker socks* can be provided and should be worn at all times when the prosthesis is not being used for the first year postop.

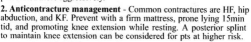

Other limb shaping options include the *immediate postoperative-fitting prosthesis* (IPOP), the *rigid removable dressing*, and cylindrical elastic bandages (e.g., Compressor-Grip and TuboGrip). *Scar mobilization* massage should be instituted as soon as tolerated to help prevent adherence of the scar to the underlying soft tissues and bone. Once the sutures are removed, the massage can be performed more aggressively.

2. Anticontracture management - Common contractures are HF, hip abduction, and KF. Prevent with a firm mattress, prone lying 15min tid, and promoting knee extension while resting. A posterior splint to maintain knee extension can be considered for pts at higher risk.

3. Pre-prosthetic and prosthetic training - Hip AROM and strengthening exercises are key. A good test to determine cardiovascular tolerance for prosthesis use is ambulation with a walker (w/o a prosthesis). Prosthetic gait training should begin with parallel bars and progress to walkers or canes. Crutches should be avoided since they promote poor gait patterns. The *definitive prosthesis* is usually created at 3-6mos.

Reference: **1**. **Garrison SJ**: *Handbook of PM&R Basics*. JB Lippincott, 1995. Figure courtesy of **Garrison SJ**: *Handbook of PM&R Basics*. JB Lippincott, 1995.

34

C. Transtibial (TT) Prosthetics

1. Socket designs

The socket connects the residual limb to the rest of the prosthesis and plays an important role in the transfer of body weight to the ground.

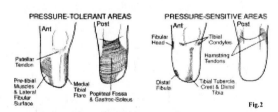

Fig.1

Above: Total contact socket.

The patellar tendon bearing (PTB) socket is an old term for the *total contact socket*. The patellar tendon actually only bears a moderate load. Weight is distributed over many areas (see "pressure-tolerant areas" in Fig. 2 below), but not over the bony prominences.

The *Icelandic Scandinavian New York (ISNY) socket* has an outer rigid frame and an inner flexible frame. The outer rigid frame has windows which provide additional local pressure relief. The durability of the ISNY socket, however, is suboptimal. The transparent *total surface-bearing socket* is less frequently used than the total contact or ISNY sockets.

For any socket, soft inserts made of polyethylene foam or silicone gel provide extra protection, e.g., for cases of PVD or extensive scarring. The inserts, however, reduce the intimacy of contact between the limb and prosthesis, which is important for proprioception. A soft foam distal end discourages verrucous hyperplasia formation.

Above: Pressure-tolerant/sensitive areas in the transtibial total contact socket.
Fig.1 courtesy of **Tan J**: *Practical Manual of PM&R*. Mosby, 1998. **Fig.2** courtesy of **Braddom R**, ed.: *PM&R*. WB Saunders, 1996.

2. Selected suspension options

Differential pressure (silicone suction with shuttle lock)⇨
A flexible, molded silicone liner is rolled directly onto the residual limb and secured to the socket with a pin. This provides optimal suspension and proprioception, but requires stable limb volumes and good hand dexterity for donning/doffing.

Anatomic - A *brim suspension* is an extension of the socket over the femoral epicondyles. This design is easy to don/doff, provides mediolateral knee stability, and is useful for short limb lengths.

The *supracondylar cuff* clips on above the epicondyles and is a common suspension option. This design is not indicated in pts with very short residual limbs or with mediolateral knee instability. A supracondylar cuff with fork strap and waist belt suspension adds additional stability for very active pts, e.g., manual laborers.

Sleeve - An elastic sleeve can serve as a primary or secondary suspension via longitudinal tension and negative pressure during swing phase. It can provide additional security for short residual limbs, when mediolateral knee stability is questionable, or when hyperextension control is required.

Figure courtesy of **Tan J**: *Practical Manual of PM&R*. Mosby, 1998.

3. Selected foot-ankle assembly options

a. *Solid ankle cushioned heel (SACH) foot* - SACH feet are light, durable, inexpensive, and stable. The soft heel simulates plantarflexion during heel strike. They are the most commonly used prosthetic foot and well suited for flat, level surfaces.

b. *Single-axis foot* - These feet are heavier but less durable than SACH feet. They are most commonly used for transfemoral amputees, i.e., when knee stability is desired (a quick foot flat improves knee stability). Only sagittal axis movement is allowed.

c. *Multi-axis foot* (Greissinger, Endolite Multiflex, SAFE II, TruStep) - The multi-axis foot allows plantar/dorsiflexion, inversion/ eversion, and rotation, which improve balance and coordination. It provides good shock absorption and is good for uneven ground, but is heavy, costly, and prone to need relatively frequent adjustments or repairs.

d. *Dynamic elastic response (DER) foot* (Seattle Light, Carbon Copy II, Quantum Foot, Flex-Foot, SpringLite) - These feet were formerly called "energy-storing feet," but they have *not* demonstrated a reduction in the energy cost or rate of energy expenditure during level walking, compared to the SACH foot[1]. They may, however, be more efficient than other feet at higher speeds. Geriatric amputees benefit from the light weight of these feet.

Reference: **1**. Torburn L, Perry J: Energy expenditure during ambulation in dysvascular and traumatic BKAs: a comparison of 5 prosthetic feet. *J Rehabil Res Dev* 1995;32:111-9. Figures courtesy of **Tan J**: *Practical Manual of PM&R*. Mosby, 1998.

D. Transfemoral (TF) Prosthetics

1. Traditional socket designs

TF sockets are often fitted in slight (5°) flexion and adduction to put stretch on the hip extensors and abductors and give them a mechanical advantage.

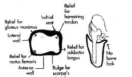

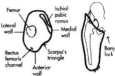

Quadrilateral design ⇑

This ischial-gluteal weight bearing, *narrow anteroposterior* design was originally designed by Inman and Eberhart at UC Berkeley in the 1950s. It has 4 sides and 4 corners. It is easy to make and fit but less stable for shorter residual limbs and less comfortable when sitting than the ischial containment design.

Ischial containment design ⇑

A "bony lock" incorporates the ischial tuberosity, pubic ramus, and greater trochanter. The posterior rim provides ischial-gluteal weight bearing and is contoured for the ischial tuberosity and gluteal muscles. These features improve stability, particularly for shorter residual limbs. The *narrow mediolateral* design also provides a more efficient energy cost of ambulation than the narrow AP design at high speeds.

The normal shape normal alignment (NSNA) and contoured adducted trochanteric-controlled alignment method (CAT-CAM) are 2 narrow M-L designs.

Figures courtesy of **Tan J**: *Practical Manual of PM&R*. Mosby, 1998.

2. Selected suspension options

Suction - Subatmospheric socket pressure maintains prosthetic attachment during swing phase. The sock bandage is pulled through a one-way valve hole. Its use is indicated in active amputees with well-shaped, non-fluctuating residual limbs.

Silesian belt or bandage - A belt attaches from the socket at the greater trochanter and wraps around the opposite iliac crest.

⇦**Total elastic suspension (belt)** (TES) - This elastic neoprene belt wraps around the proximal prosthesis and waist, enhancing rotational control. It retains body heat and has limited durability.

Pelvic band and belt suspension - A rigid belt is connected to a metal hip joint on the lateral side of the socket. Indicated for improving rotational and M-L pelvic stability in obese pts with significant redundant tissue or weak abductors with short or poorly shaped amputations. It is heavy and bulky, and tends to interfere with sitting.

3. Selected knee components, key features

Single-axis or constant friction - This knee is durable and inexpensive, but the cadence is fixed, or else the swing phase will be asymmetric. Stability is poor. It is indicated for level surfaces.

Stance control or safety - The safety knee cannot be flexed during weight bearing, which provides stability during stance phase. It is a common initial prosthesis used in geriatrics, general debility and poor hip control. It allows ambulation on uneven surfaces. A delayed swing phase is noted, as full unloading is needed to flex the knee.

⇦**Polycentric** - This typically has a 4-bar linkage design and a shifting instantaneous center of rotation that remains behind the GRF, providing increased stability during stance phase. The center of rotation moves proximally and posteriorly to the anatomic knee's. Cosmesis is excellent, especially during sitting, but polycentrics are heavy, costly, and require high maintenance. It is indicated for knee disarticulations and short TF amputees.

Fluid controlled (pneumatic or oil) - The design uses a piston in a fluid-filled cylinder, which provides automatic swing phase control at variable cadences. It provides a smooth and natural gait, but is heavy, costly, and requires high maintenance.

Manual locking or fixed lock - The knee of last resort, this design provides the ultimate in stability. The gait, however, is awkward and energy consuming.

See p.35 for foot-ankle options. Figures courtesy of **Braddom R.** ed.: *PM&R.* WB Saunders, 1996.

E. Selected Post-Amputation Complications

1. **Phantom pain** - This can begin to develop at any time post-amputation, even yrs later. A survey of 255 community-based lower limb amputees reported phantom sensations in 79% and phantom pain in 72% at 6mos post-amputation, although many described their phantom pain as episodic and not particularly bothersome[1]. Jensen reported phantom pain to be significantly more frequent in pts with long-lasting pre-amputation pain and with pain immediately prior to amputation[2]. In the same study, pre-amputation pain had similar location and character to phantom pain in 36% of pts immediately post-amputation, but in only 10% later in the course[2].

Different treatment regimens have had varying success in the literature, including stump massage, stump US, stump wrapping, TENS, β-blockers, anticonvulsants (e.g., gabapentin), low dose tricyclic antidepressants (e.g., amitriptyline), antiarrhythmics (e.g., mexilitine), calcitonin, topical analgesics, trigger point injections, chemical sympathectomy, and anesthetic procedures. Regular use of the prosthesis can also reduce phantom pains. Narcotics are generally not recommended.

2. **Choke syndrome** - Distal limb edema and painful *verrocous hyperplasia* may develop due to proximal limb pressure and a lack of total contact with the prosthesis. An underlying vascular disorder is usually present. Treatment involves adding a distal pad to the socket, correcting the suspension, removing proximal pressure, and/or refitting the socket.

References: **1. Ehde DM:** Chronic phantom sensations, phantom pain, residual limb pain, and other regional pain after lower limb amputation. *Arch PMR* 2000;81:1039-44. **2. Jensen TS:** Immediate and long-term phantom limb pain in amputees-incidence, clinical characteristics, and relationship to preamputation limb pain. *Pain* 1985;21:267-78.

F. Prosthetic Gait Analysis

1. Relationship of amputation level(s) with energy cost & speed

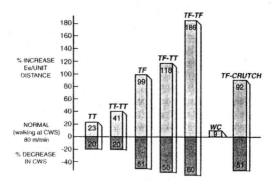

CWS = comfortable walking speed, which corresponds to the minimum energy cost per unit distance. Ee (energy expenditure)/unit distance and CWS for amputees using prostheses are compared in the figure above to able-bodied subjects at a CWS of 80 m/min (~3mi/hr). The energy cost of ambulation at CWS for able-bodied subjects is 4.3kcal/min.

Figure courtesy of **Gonzalez EG**, ed.: *Downey and Darling's The Physiological Basis of Rehabilitation Medicine*, 3rd ed. Butterworth-Heinemann, 2001.

2. Causes of stance phase problems

Excessive trunk extension/lumbar lordosis during stance phase - A poorly shaped posterior wall may cause a pt to forwardly rotate their pelvis for pressure relief, with compensatory trunk extension. Other causes include insufficient initial flexion built into socket, HF contracture, and weak hip extensors.

Foot slap - Foot slap may be noted with a transfemoral locked-knee prosthesis if the foot is posteriorly placed or if socket flexion is excessive.

Knee buckling/instability - Causes include knee axis too anterior, insufficient PF, failure to limit DF, weak hip extensors, hard heel, large HF contracture, and posteriorly-placed foot. Stability is achieved with a plantarflexed foot, a soft heel (i.e., SACH), or a more anteriorly placed foot.

Lateral bending - Causes include a prosthesis that is too short, insufficient lateral wall, abducted socket, abduction contracture, and poor amputee balance.

Vaulting - Vaulting of the non-prosthetic limb may be due to a prosthesis that is too long, too much knee friction, or poor suspension.

Whip - A whip is an abrupt rotation of the heel occurring at the end of stance phase as the knee of a transfemoral prosthesis is flexed to begin swing. If the heel moves medially, it is a medial whip; if laterally, a lateral whip. Causes include improper rotatory alignment of the knee axis, a knee axis not parallel to the floor, or flabby muscles about the femur with the prosthesis rotating freely within the underlying soft tissue.

3. Causes of swing phase problems

Abducted gait - Causes include a prosthesis that is too long, an abduction contracture, or a medial socket wall encroaching the groin.

Circumducted gait - Causes include a prosthesis that is too long, too much knee friction making it difficult to bend the knee during swing-through, or an abduction contracture.

Excessive heel rise - Causes include insufficient knee friction or excessive KF moment (i.e., posterior foot or insufficient PF at heel strike).

Foot drag - Causes include inadequate suspension, a prosthesis that is too long, insufficient HF or KF, or weak PF of the non-prosthetic limb.

Terminal swing impact - Insufficient knee friction may cause the amputee to deliberately and forcibly extend knee.

G. Upper Limb Prosthetics

Unilateral amputees typically learn to perform most ADLs with their intact hand. B/l amputees often use their feet for many ADLs. Functional UEx prostheses should be prescribed for highly motivated pts with realistic expectations. Residual limb shaping with bandages may be required for 1-2mos before prosthetic fitting. If fitting is not performed within a 3-6mos window after unilateral amputation, long-term prosthesis use is infrequently seen.

1. Transradial (TR) prosthetics

Body-powered prostheses with hook hands are typically prescribed for manual laborers (the typical pt who is going to suffer a traumatic UEx amputation in the first place). Lifting up to 20-30lbs can be expected. Longer residual limbs provide more lever arm, more pronation/supination, and are better suited for heavy labor. Myoelectric prostheses are often appropriate for relatively sedentary amputees.

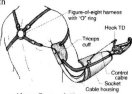

Above: Commonly seen components in a TR prosthesis.

2. Transhumeral (TH) prosthetics

Longer residual limbs (up to 90% of original/expected length) are preferred. Function is usually much poorer than with a TR. A key difference for TH prostheses users is the need for an elbow unit. Harnessing and control systems are also different. Lifting up to 10-15lbs can be expected (more with a shoulder saddle). Length estimates for b/l TH amputees are 19% of pt height for the upper arm and 21% for the forearm component.

Figure courtesy of **Grabois M**: *PM&R: The Complete Approach.* Blackwell Publishing, 1999.

3. Functional terminal devices (TD)

The TD is the most important functional part of the UEx prosthesis. The proximal limb/prosthesis essentially functions to position the TD in space. Body-powered *voluntary opening (VO)* split-hooks are the most common and practical TDs. Prehensile force is predetermined by the # of rubber bands in place (each provides ~1lb pinch force). Up to 10 bands can be used (typical non-amputee ♂ pinch force is 15-20lbs). *Voluntary closing (VC)* TDs provide better control of closing pressure, but active effort is required to maintain closure of the TD or items may be dropped.

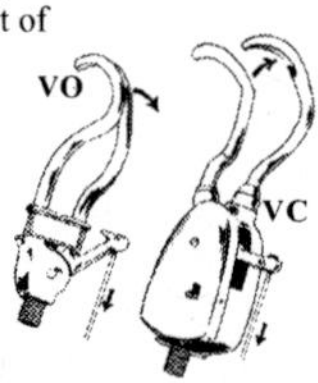

Fig.1

Myoelectric hands offer spherical/palmar grasp with grip forces higher than body-powered TDs. They can have a life-like appearance but are relatively fragile. 2-site 2-fxn controllers use different muscles to open and close the TD, while 1-site 2-fxn controllers use weak versus strong contractions of the same muscle to operate the TD.

4. UEx prosthetic systems basic needs[1]

| | Control | | Shape | |
	body pwr	myoelectric	hook	hand
Function				
fine tip prehension	-	-	✓	-
cylindrical grip (large diameter)	-	-	-	✓
cylindrical grip (sm diameter)	-	-	✓	-
high grip force	-	✓	-	-
delicate grip force	-	✓	-	-
hook and pull	-	-	✓	-
pushing/holding down	-	-	-	✓
ruggedness	✓	-	✓	-
Comfort				
low weight	✓	-	✓	-
harness comfort	-	✓	-	-
low effort	-	✓	-	-
Reliability/convenience	✓	-	✓	-
Cosmesis	-	-	-	✓
Low cost	✓	-	-	-

Reference: **1. Dillingham T**, specialist ed.: *Rehabilitation of the Injured Combatant Part IV.* Office of the Surgeon General, Dept. of Army, 1998. **Fig.1** courtesy of **Kottke F**, ed.: *Krusen's Handbook of PM&R*, 4th ed. WB Saunders, 1990.

5. Other components

The most common prosthetic *wrist* is the *friction wrist*, which allows passive pronation/supination but rotates when holding heavy objects. B/l amputees require at least one mechanical spring-assisted *flexion wrist* for access to the body midline. Most TH prosthetic **elbows** have an *alternator lock*, which alternately locks and unlocks with the same movement. With the elbow unlocked, body movements will flex or extend the elbow using a cable; when locked, the same cable operates the TD.

The traditional suspension employs straps and cables, with a double-walled **socket** for optimal fit. The outer wall is rigid and connects to other components; the inner wall must fit with the residual limb precisely or else the prosthesis may fail. The *suction socket* can provide self-suspension w/o straps and ideally is preferred for the TH amputee. The *Munster supracondylar socket* provides self-suspension for a very short TR or elbow disarticulation by encasing the humeral condyles and can be used for externally powered prostheses. Proper fit of the Munster socket, however, precludes full elbow extension.

The **body harness** uses cables to allow body motion and effort to operate prosthetic components. The *figure-of-8*, generally for a short TR or more proximal amputation, also holds the socket firmly in place, usually with an elbow hinge and half-arm cuff or triceps pad. The *figure-of-9*, generally for a long TR or wrist disarticulation, requires a self-suspending socket but is more comfortable than the 8. The *shoulder saddle with chest strap* frees the opposite shoulder and relieves the pressure caused by the axillary loop of the 8. Heavy loads are better tolerated, but donning is difficult and cosmesis is inferior.

6. Body-powered prosthesis control

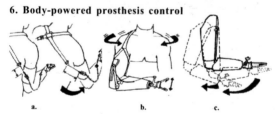

a.   b.   c.

a. Glenohumeral forward flexion (TR, TH) - This natural movement provides excellent power and reach and can activate the TD or flex an elbow joint.

b. Biscapular ABDuction (Forequarter, shoulder disarticulation, TH, TR) - This movement can activate a TD, but the TD must stay relatively stationary. Generated forces are relatively weak.

c. GH depression, extension, ABDuction (TH) - This movement locks or unlocks an elbow, but may be unnatural for some users and difficult to master.

d. Scapular elevation (not pictured) - This locks or unlocks the elbow and is easy to master. It requires a waist belt.

e. Chest expansion/scapular ADDuction (not pictured) - This locks or unlocks the elbow. It is an awkward motion, but does not interfere with TD operations.

Body-powered prosthesis control figures courtesy of **Northwestern University Orthotics and Prosthetics Center**, modified with permission.

VI. ORTHOTICS

A. Spinal Orthotics

1. Selected rostral spinal orthoses

The *Philadelphia collar*, a popular cervical orthosis, is indicated for stable mid-cervical bony or ligamentous injuries. It is also frequently used after weaning off a more rigid orthosis. Rotation and lateral bending are not as well controlled as flexion and extension. The Aspen, Miami, and Malibu collars are popular alternatives because of their padding and comfort.

The *SOMI*, named for its points of attachment (sternal-occipital mandibular immobilizer) is useful for bed-ridden pts because of its lack of posterior uprights. Its stabilizing effects are similar to other poster orthoses, but donning/doffing are relatively easier.

The *Halo* vest (right) is frequently used to treat cervical fxs and dislocations and is the only option between C0 and C2. The rigid headpiece, secured to the skull by four pins, is bolted to four posters that connect to a rigid polyethylene vest or plaster cast. Studies have shown that there is some movement between cervical segments (snaking phenomenon) and that PT does not increase motion between segments[1]. Vital capacity may be limited. The shoulder should not be abducted >90°. Pin care with saline+soap is required bid-tid. H_2O_2, povidone-iodine, and hypochlorite are all associated with more infections than saline+soap[2].

The Halo is typically worn for 12wks. Complications include pin loosening, infection, ring migration, pressure sores, and pin scars.

The *thermoplastic Minerva body jacket* is a lightweight alternative to the Halo in selected pts. It restricts below C2 similarly to the Halo w/o the need for pins, but cannot be used for instability between the occiput to C2 where a Halo may be the only choice.

2. Effects of selected orthoses on cervical motion

(occiput to C7) in percentage of mean normal motion allowed[3]

	Flex/extension	Lateral-bending	Rotation
Normal	100	100	100
Soft collar	74.2	92.3	82.6
Philadelphia collar	28.9	66.4	43.7
SOMI brace	27.7	65.6	33.6
4-poster brace	20.6	45.9	27.1
Yale C-T brace	12.8	50.5	18.2
Minerva jacket	14.0	15.5	0
Halo device	4.0-11.7	4.0-8.4	1.0-2.4

References: 1. Lind B: Forces and motions across the neck in pts treated with halo-vest. *Spine* 1988;13:162-7. 2. Olson RS: HALO skeletal traction pinsite care: towards developing a standard of care. *Rehabil Nursing* 1996;21:243-6. 3. Johnson RM: Cervical orthosis: a study comparing their effectiveness in restricting cervical motion in normal subjects. *JBJS (Am)* 1977;59:332-9. Philadelphia collar figure courtesy of Redford J. ed.: *Orthotics Etcetera*, 3rd ed. Williams & Wilkins, 1986.

3. Selected nonrigid truncal orthoses

The *trochanteric belt* (A) is used for SI joint-related pain and for healing pelvic fxs.

The *sacroiliac belt* (B) provides kinesthetic feedback to maintain a neutral pelvis and some SI joint stability. It is used for traumatic or post-partum SI separation. A perineal strap reduces rostral migration.

The *lumbosacral belt* (C) is often prescribed for LBP associated with degenerative disc disorders, postural fatigue, OA and other conditions where abdominal compression is thought to relieve pain by decreasing spinal load. Support for its use, however, is not strongly documented in the literature. As with most truncal orthoses, PT should be prescribed to prevent truncal atrophy.

The *lumbosacral corset* (D) extends more rostrally and caudally to provide a more cosmetic contour than the LS belt, but the extra material may be uncomfortable in warm weather. Functionally, it is similar to the belt. Side lacing with pull straps provide a 4-1 mechanical advantage, so that each pound of force applied to the strap transfers 4lbs of pressure over the abdomen.

The *thoracolumbar corset* (E) is helpful for the control of pain in generalized osteoporosis, metastatic malignancy, myeloma, and thoracic OA. Obese individuals typically derive *more* benefit from corsets than thin persons because of snugger fit.

4. Selected rigid truncal orthoses

The *anterior hyperextension (Jewett) orthosis* (F) uses the 3-point pressure system (manubrium sternum, midback, pubic symphysis) to allow extension, but limit flexion. Although light-weight, comfort is suboptimal due to the high pressure at each area. It is indicated primarily after surgical stabilization of lower thoracic or upper lumbar fractures and is not recommended in osteoporosis because of the risk of posterior element fxs.

The *LS extension-lateral control (Williams) orthosis* (G) is a short dynamic brace that allows flexion and is useful for spondylolysis and spondylolisthesis. It is not used with compression fxs.

The Chairback brace is a *LS flexion-extension-lateral control orthosis* often prescribed for LBP and disk herniation since it decreases lumbar lordosis and increases intraabdominal pressure. It is sometimes used as a prognosticator in candidates considering spinal fusion.

The *TLS flexion-extension control (Taylor) orthosis* (H) is primarily used for kyphosis 2° to stable osteoporotic fxs.

The *custom-molded TLS body jacket (clam-shell) orthosis* provides the most lower truncal immobilization. It is indicated for postsurgical thoracolumbar fixation and is effective as rostral as T8.

The *Knight brace* (I) provides support that is similar to the Chairback. The Knight brace, however, has lateral bars and a corset that only covers the anterior trunk.

Truncal orthotics figures courtesy of **Redford J**, ed.: *Orthotics Etcetera*, 3rd ed. Williams & Wilkins, 1986.

B. UEx Orthotics

1. Selected orthoses

Shoulder abduction stabilizer ⇨
(Airplane splint) - Protects the shoulder from adduction contracture (e.g., axillary burn, post shoulder surgery) and relieves tension on the deltoid and rotator cuff. It is not well tolerated.

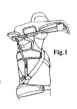

Fig.1

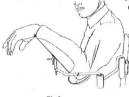

Fig.2

⇦ **Mobile arm support (MAS)**
(Balanced forearm orthosis) - The forearm trough is mounted to a swivel mechanism that supports the weight of the upper limb against gravity. It allows those with profound proximal weakness but some preserved active elbow flexion and shoulder motion, e.g., C5 SCI, to functionally use their hand. Hand orthoses with attachments for utensils are often used. Some C4s may benefit from a MAS. Powered versions also exist.

Wrist-extensor finger-flexion orthosis ⇨
(Rancho flexor-hinge tenodesis splint) - Using the traditional tenodesis orthosis, a C6 tetra with ≥3+ strength in the wrist extensors and good DIP ROM can achieve a passive 3-point chuck grip with active wrist extension. Shoulder driven finger flexion is also possible. C4 and C5 tetras may benefit from a electric power-assisted tenodesis orthosis.

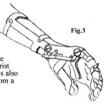

Fig.3

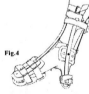

Fig.4

⇦ **Pancake splint**
- This is used to counteract wrist and finger flexion contracture, e.g., hemiplegia. A bent dorsal steel bar applies additional extension force against wrist flexion. This orthosis is restrictive and is often used as a night splint for stretching. Daytime use may be acceptable for patients without functional hand use.

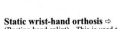

Fig.5

Static wrist-hand orthosis ⇨
(Resting hand splint) - This is used to rest an injured hand, prevent contracture, or stretch a contracture. The arches of the hand are maintained, and the thumb is kept abducted.

Wrist extension hinge/spring assist ⇨ long opponens orthosis

(Rancho long opponens splint) - This dynamic orthosis has a hinged wrist joint and a rubber band that provides extension assist. The distal portion of the orthosis supports the thumb during opposition, and maintains the palmar transverse arch. Some orthoses have slots for the attachment of utensils, e.g., spoons, pencils.

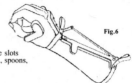

Fig.6

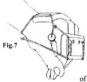

Fig.7

⇦Knuckle bender orthosis

This device is a dynamic MCP flexion hand orthosis, which attempts to reverse the effects of extension contractures of the MCP joints. A reverse knuckle bender exerts force against the palmar surface to reverse the effects of MCP flexion.

Dorsal MCP extension stop orthosis ⇨

The "lumbrical bar" is designed to enhance the extension of the interphalangeal joints by the long extensor muscles in an intrinsic minus hand (e.g., clawhand due to median and ulnar neuropathy).

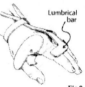

Lumbrical bar

Fig.8

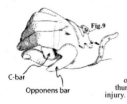

Fig.9

⇦ C-bar short opponens orthosis

The opponens bar prevents a weak thumb (e.g., median neuropathy) from extending inadvertently. The C-bar maintains thumb (palmar) abduction. Together they position the thumb in opposition to the other digits to facilitate three-jaw chuck pinch. This orthosis can also can provide rest to the thumb in CMC arthritis or collateral ligament injury.

C-bar

Opponens bar

Modified utensils ⇨

A built-up handle (A) helps those with weak grips to hold their utensils more firmly. Spoon or fork shafts can be bent to accommodate persons with reduced ROM in the upper limb (B). A universal cuff utensil holder (C) and rocker knife (D) are some tools that can be useful for tetraplegics or others with limited intrinsic hand function.

Fig.10

Figs.1,2,3,4,6,7,10 courtesy of **Redford J**, ed.: *Orthotics Etcetera*, 3rd ed. Williams & Wilkins, 1986. **Fig.5** courtesy of **Paget SA**, ed.: *Manual of Rheumatology and Outpatient Orthopedic Disorders*. LWW, 2000. **Figs.8,9** courtesy of **Kottke F**, ed.: *Krusen's Handbook of PM&R*. 4th ed. WB Saunders, 1990.

C. LEx Orthotics

1. Ankle foot orthoses (AFO)

a. Thermoplastic molded AFOs (Fig.1)

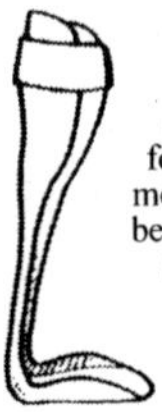

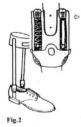

Plastic offers the advantages of light weight, cosmesis, low expense, and the ability to interchange shoes. Sensate limbs with no or stabilized edema are prerequisite since the trim lines may cause pressure damage. Some general issues to consider include: 1) the foot component should extend at least beyond the metatarsal heads; 2) AFOs prescribed for foot drop should be just rigid enough to allow for toe clearance (increased rigidity, however, can exacerbate knee instability at heel strike); 3) the calf shell should end proximally 1" below the fibular head to avoid peroneal n. damage; 4) for unilateral AFO users, shoes that are a 1/2 size larger on the AFO side may be required to accommodate the AFO (some higher-end department stores may allow this kind of sale).

Fig.1

The *posterior leaf spring* (not pictured) simulates a posterior spring dual metal upright AFO (**Fig.2**), preventing foot drop but allowing some plantarflexion at heel strike. It does not provide mediolateral stability due to its low ankle trim line.

b. Double metal upright AFO

Two metal uprights are connected proximally to a calf band with a rigid posterior and soft anterior. Hinge joints at the distal end control ankle motion. A stirrup with sole plate attaches the AFO to the shoe. Metal AFOs are not used as frequently as in the past, but are indicated for excessive edema, fluctuating edema, or for the insensate limb. They are less likely to break at the foot-ankle junction as strength is superior to plastic AFOs. Placing different components (e.g., pins, springs) into the ankle channel(s) may assist or limit motions occurring at the ankle.

⇔ **AFO dual channel component options**
(posterior spring and anterior pin shown on left)

anterior pin	- limits ADF beyond setting of pin
anterior spring	- not used (no spring strong enough to assist APF)
posterior pin	- limits APF beyond setting of pin
posterior spring	- assists ADF, limits some APF

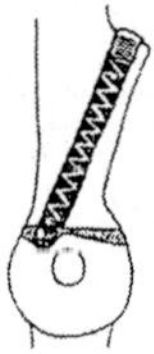

Fig.2

Klenzak joint

Fig.3

A spring loaded into the single posterior channel of the *Klenzak joint* (**Fig.3**) provides ADF assist.

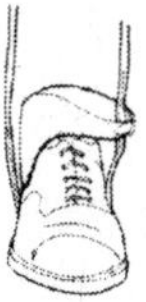

T-Strap

The t-strap is used with double metal upright AFOs to enhance medial or lateral stability at the ankle. For valgus deformity or laxity, use a *medial* T-strap that attaches onto shoe over the medial malleolus and straps around the lateral upright. When cinched, this pulls the medial malleolus laterally. For varus deformity or laxity, use a *lateral* T-strap.

Fig.4

c. Patellar tendon bearing (PTB) AFO ⇨

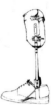

The proximal component is designed to support weight on the patellar tendon and tibial flares with the load being transmitted to the shoe by metal uprights. Indications include healing diabetic foot ulcers, tibial fractures, post-op ankle fusions, painful heel conditions (e.g., calcaneal fractures), or AVN of the foot or ankle.

d. AFO options for selected clinical conditions

Fig.5

Foot drop - Options include a posterior leaf spring AFO or a double metal upright AFO with Klenzak joint. A double metal upright AFO with a posterior stop at 90° is another option; however, the lack of plantarflexion during early stance phase may destabilize the knee.

Foot drop and weak quadriceps - An AFO with a posterior stop at 90° addresses the foot drop, but may further destabilize a weak knee (e.g., weak quads) because APF is precluded during early stance phase. The posterior stop should be set, instead, at the minimal level required to clear the foot during swing phase. Alternatives include a Klenzak joint or posterior spring, which allow plantarflexion during stance phase.

Foot drop and weak plantarflexors - A solid plastic AFO or double metal upright AFO with anterior and posterior stops can be prescribed.

Mediolateral instability - On double metal uprights, t-straps can be used. For plastic AFOs, the trim line at the ankle can be cut more anteriorly.

Plantar spasticity - An option is an AFO with a posterior stop and a sole plate extending beyond the metatarsal heads (to improve the lever arm against the spasticity).

Pain with ankle motion - A solid AFO or AFO with anterior and posterior stops can reduce ankle movement (and pain).

Weak plantarflexors - An option is an AFO with an anterior stop at 5° of dorsiflexion and a sole plate extending to metatarsal heads (so the shoe can pivot over the metatarsal heads, simulating push off). This will also stabilize the knee during push off.

Further readings **1**. **Sarno JE**: Prescription considerations for plastic below-knee orthoses. *Arch PMR* 1971;52:503-10. **2**. **Lehmann JF**: Biomechanics of AFO:Prescription and design *Arch PMR* 1979;60:200-7. **Figs.1,2** courtesy of **Wu KK**: *Foot Orthoses: Principles and Clinical Practice.* Williams & Wilkins, 1990. **Figs.3,4,5** courtesy of **Redford J**, ed.: *Orthotics Etcetera*, 3rd ed. Williams & Wilkins, 1986.

2. Knee-ankle-foot orthoses (KAFO)

KAFOs provide knee, ankle, and subtalar joint stability. A KAFO might be used unilaterally for polio patients and bilaterally for SCI pts. For low thoracic and high lumbar SCI pts, the use of posterior and anterior stops at the ankle reduces energy consumption. Shown at right is a double metal upright KAFO with dual thigh bands and knee joints. The distal portion is similar to an AFO.

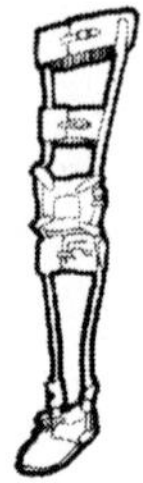

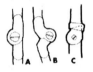

Knee joints

Fig.1

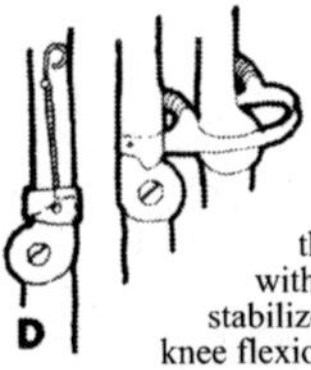

Free motion (A) - Free motion knees can allow unlimited flexion and extension but hyperextension is usually prevented by a stop. It is indicated for genu recurvatum or mediolateral instability.

Fig.2

Offset knee (B) - The hinge is posterior to the axis of rotation so that the GRF is relatively anterior, which stabilizes the knee during early stance. Free knee flexion is allowed during swing and sitting is unimpeded. This knee joint is *not* to be used with a knee or hip contracture or PF stop.

Drop-ring (C) - Gravity brings the ring(s) into the locked position when the user stands erect with knee(s) in full extension. Ambulation may be stabilized. The rings can be manually released to allow knee flexion during sitting.

Pawl lock with bail release (D) - A spring loaded projection (pawl) locks both medial and lateral joints. The semicircular lever (bail), which attaches posteriorly, is easily engaged to unlock both joints.

The **Craig-Scott orthosis** (CSO) is a light, easily donnable KAFO for complete SCI pts with injuries at L1 or above. It can be used for standing and/or ambulation. The components include double metal uprights, a knee joint with pawl locks and bail control, a posterior thigh band, a hinged pretibial band, ankle joints set at slight (5-10°) dorsiflexion (BiCAAL, Bi-Channel Adjustable Ankle Lock with adjustable anterior and posterior pins), and a shoe with a cushion heel and T-shaped foot plate. Hip stability is achieved by maintaining the trunk in extension so that the GRF passes behind the hip. Ambulation is typically achieved via a swing-to or swing-thru gait with forearm crutches.

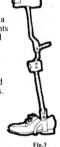

Fig.3

Figs.1,2,3 courtesy of **Tan J**: *Practical Manual of PM&R*. Mosby, 1998.

3. Other LEx orthoses

Reciprocating gait orthosis (RGO), adult-type -
Special cables on this b/l HKAFO transfer hip flexion
forces on one side to hip extension on the other and
vice versa to provide a more "natural" appearing
reciprocal gait pattern than the CSO. B/l HF is
precluded by the cables during ambulation, but this
mechanism can be released to allow for sitting.
Donning and doffing, however, are difficult, and
energy expenditure using the RGO with a
reciprocating gait is higher than a swing-through
pattern with the CSO.

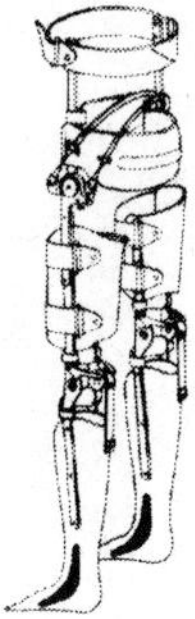

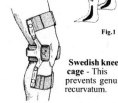

Fig.1

**Infrapatellar (Cho-pat)
strap KO** - This KO is a
foam-padded strap that
encircles the knee
immediately below the
patella. It is worn
during periods of
activity to help control **Fig.2**
tracking of the patella in
patellofemoral disorders.

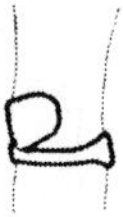

**Swedish knee
cage** - This
prevents genu
recurvatum.

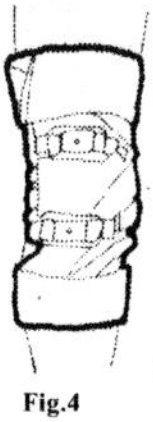

Fig.3

**Lenox Hill
derotation orthosis**
- It is used for post
ACL surgery, ACL
tears, and ACL
deficient knees and
prevents anterior
translation of tibia on
femur.

Fig.4

Moonboot (not pictured)
- The moonboot locks the
ankle into neutral to
provide stability and
prevent painful ankle
motion. Its rocker-bottom
sole helps to distribute
weight bearing more
evenly over the entire
foot.

UCBL (U. Calif. Biomechanics
Lab) - This rigid plastic orthosis
is fabricated over a plaster mold of
the foot held in maximum manual
correction. It realigns flexible flat
feet (pes valgus), especially in
runners. It encompasses the heel
with rigid walls to
stabilize the
intertarsal/
TMT
joints.

Heel cup - This rigid plastic
cup covers the
posterior plantar
surface, reducing
lateral
calcaneal
shift. It
is used
for flexible
pes planus.

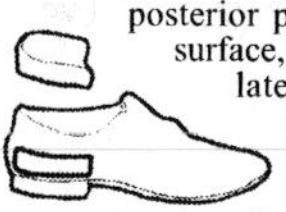

Fig.6

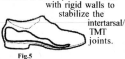

Fig.5

Fig.1 courtesy of **Redford J**, ed.: *Orthotics Etcetera*, 3rd ed. Williams & Wilkins,
1986. **Figs.2,4,5,6** courtesy of **Tan J**: *Practical Manual of PM&R*. Mosby, 1998. **Fig.3**
courtesy of **DeLisa J**, ed.: *Rehabilitation Medicine: Principles and Practice*, 3rd ed.
Lippincott-Raven, 1998.

50

4. Shoes

a. Basic shoe types and parts

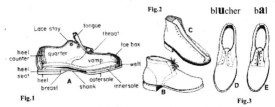

Fig.1

Fig.2

bl**u**cher b**a**l

Fig.3

A. Basic parts of the *Oxford* (low quarter) shoe. **B.** *High quarter* ("high-top" or chukka) - The apices of the malleoli are covered. There is increased sensory feedback and decreased pistoning of the shoe (decreases chafing), but no significant mediolateral stability. **C.** The *convalescent* shoe is a special type of Blucher shoe worn after surgery or for the ankylosed foot. The lacing extends to the toes, which provides the easiest mode of entry for a foot that cannot be plantarflexed. **D.** *Blucher* - The open throat design (the tongue is continuous with vamp) allows easy entry of the foot. (Mnemonic: remember that the top of the letter "u" in Blucher is "open", whereas the "a" in Bal is "closed.") **E.** *Bal* (balmoral) - The closed throat design is usually prescribed when there is no problem in the forefoot.

Fig.1 courtesy of **DeLisa J**, ed.: *Rehabilitation Medicine: Principles and Practice*, 3rd ed. Lippincott-Raven, 1998. **Figs.2,3** courtesy of **Redford J**, ed.: *Orthotics Etcetera*, 3rd ed. Williams & Wilkins, 1986.

b. Common shoe modifications

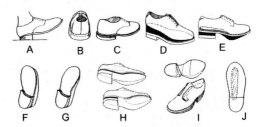

A. The *cushioned heel* simulates ankle plantar flexion and stabilizes the knee and is often used with a rocker bar for a more natural gait. **B.** An *external heel flare* can be used to resist either varus ankle motion (with a lateral flare) or valgus motion (with a medial flare). The flare can also partially unload the medial compartment of the knee (with a lateral flare) or the lateral compartment (with a medial flare). **C.** *External heel wedge.* **D.** *Combination external sandwich-elevation* of heel and sole. **E.** *Shoe lift with rocker bar at sole.* The rocker bottom relieves pressure from the metatarsal (MT) heads and assists in rollover when the plantarflexors are weak. The Denver bar is a leather MT support used for similar purposes. **F.** The medial wedge of the *Thomas (orthopedic) heel* extends anteriorly under the navicular bone and provides support to the medial longitudinal arch. **G.** The *reverse Thomas (reverse orthopedic) heel* supports the lateral longitudinal arch; it is seldom used. **H.** *Combination medial sole and heel wedging* promotes foot supination and may be appropriate when too much weight is borne on the medial side, e.g., foot valgus. Lateral sole and heel wedging promotes pronation. **I.** The *lateral sole flare* helps to resist foot inversion and provides greater stability. The medial flare resists eversion. **J.** A *steel bar* is placed between the inner and outer soles to reduce anterior sole movement and stress at the MTs and phalanges. It is often used in conjunction with a rocker bottom sole.

c. Miscellaneous shoe issues[1]

For *leg lengths that are unequal*, but <0.5" different, an internal heel elevation may be sufficient; if >0.5" an external heel elevation is necessary. If >1", heel + sole elevation should be used.

For *pes plano-valgus*, the goal is to reduce eversion and to support the longitudinal arch (e.g., Thomas heel with medial high wedge, medial longitudinal arch support with cookie or scaphoid pad).

For *hallux valgus*, a shoe may be prescribed with some or all of the following features: soft vamp with broad ball and toe, relief in the vamp with cut-out or balloon patch, low heel, metatarsal or sesamoid pad, medial longitudinal arch support. The idea is to reduce pressure on the 1st MTP and hallux, to prevent forward foot slide, and to shift weight laterally.

Reference: **1.** Ragnarsson KT: Lower Extremity Orthotics, Shoes, and Gait Aids. In DeLisa J, ed.: *Rehabilitation Medicine: Principles and Practice*, 3rd ed. Lippincott-Raven, 1998. Figures courtesy of Redford J, ed.: *Orthotics Etcetera*, 3rd ed. Williams & Wilkins, 1986 and Fu F, Stone D: *Sports Injuries: Mechanisms, Prevention & Tx.* Williams & Wilkins, 1994.

E. LEx Orthotics and Gait

1. **The key concept** - Different components of the LEx (particularly the ankle-foot portion) can either promote knee flexion (possibly leading to knee instability), or promote knee extension (providing more stability, but possibly leading to genu recurvatum).

Promotes Knee Flexion	Promotes Knee Extension
Ankle dorsiflexion	Ankle plantarflexion
Limit plantar flexion (posterior stop)	Limit dorsiflexion (anterior stop)
Posterior ground reactive force	Anterior ground reactive force
Short sole shank (during toe off)	Long sole shank (during toe off)

2. **Knee stability pearls**
a. The more the knee is destabilized by the orthosis, the stronger the quads must be to prevent buckling.
b. Weak knee extensors can lead to genu recurvatum as the knee is thrown into extension to prevent buckling.

VII. WHEELCHAIR
A. Manual wheelchairs (WC)

1. Typical measurements

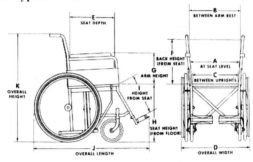

Back height (F)	self propeller, good trunk control	2" below inf. angle of scapula
	self propeller, poor trunk control	2" below scapular spine
	poor UEx strength, poor trunk control	standard (typically 16.5")
Seat width (C)	(widest point, usually hip, plus 1")	18"
Seat depth (E)	(buttock to popliteal fossa, minus 2")	16"
Seat height (H)	(popliteal fossa to floor, plus 2")	19"
WC width	18" seat width usually corresponds to 27" WC width. (Doorways need to have a clearance that is ≥ 32" wide to be ADA compliant).	
WC weight*	standard (no set definition)	~43-50 lbs
	light weight	<35 lbs
	ultra light weight (i.e., sports chairs)	<28 lbs
	heavy duty (for users >250 lbs)	45-60 lbs
Wheel size	standard	24"
	"hemi chair"	20"

*Decreasing the weight of a manual WC does not necessarily increase propulsion efficiency on level surfaces, but a difference is appreciable on uphill grades. Figure courtesy of **Redford J.** ed.: *Orthotics Etcetera*, 3rd ed. Williams & Wilkins, 1986.

2. Prescription considerations

Frame - Folding frames are easier to transport but may be heavier, less durable, and require more energy to propel. Rigid frame chairs are more durable and energy efficient during propulsion, but may be more difficult to transport.

Axle - Posterior placement is advantageous for users with poor trunk control, amputees, reclining/posterior tilt WCs, but increases turning radius, rolling resistance, and the difficulty of doing wheelies. Anterior placement decreases rolling resistance and improves maneuverability (decreased turning radius, easier wheelies), but also increases risk of tipping over backwards.

Molded plastic (mag) vs. wire-spoked wheels - Mag wheels are slightly heavier but more durable than spoked wheels. Spoked wheels are preferred in most sports chairs, but require more maintenance and are less safe for some individuals whose fingers may get caught in the spokes.

Pneumatic vs. rubber tires - Pneumatic (air-filled innertube) tires offer a comfortable ride on uneven terrain but are susceptible to going flat and have a higher resistance to propulsion. Solid rubber tires may be preferred if the WC is mostly to be used indoors (i.e., office work, hospitals, nursing homes) due to the easier propulsion and low maintenance.

Camber - Standard camber is 7° (range 3-9°). Increasing camber decreases turning radius, improves side-to-side and forward stability, decreases rolling resistance at high speeds (no effect at normal speeds), and protects user hands during sports. Disadvantages include difficulty in tight spaces due to increased overall WC width, increased tire/wheel-bearing wear, and decreased rear stability.

Handrims - Small diameter handrims (sports WCs) increase the distance covered with each stroke, but require greater force. Pegged handrims ("quad knobs") improve ease of use for tetraplegics and users with hand deformities but increase risk of trauma during attempts to stop.

Casters - Small (≤5" diameter), narrow casters are appropriate for smooth, level surfaces, and less likely to shimmy. Large (≥6" diameter), wide casters are advantageous in rougher, outdoor terrain, but have increased rolling resistance on smooth surfaces, and are more likely to shimmy.

Cushions - *Foam cushions* are lightweight and inexpensive, but are not washable and dissipate heat poorly.

Gel cushions (i.e., Jay, Jay-2) consist of a firm gel emulsion enclosed in a non-breathable plastic that provides good postural stability. They are durable, easy to maintain and clean, and offer a high capacity to dissipate skin heat buildup, but are expensive, heavy, and the contouring can interfere with transfers. The new Jay-2 has "memory," which maintains optimal configuration.

Air-filled villous cushions, such as the ROHO, consist of multiple balloon-like air cells that assure maximum skin contact and provide the best pressure relief. The design is favorable for pressure ulcer prevention or healing. These cushions are lightweight, good at heat dissipation, and easy to clean and transport, but expensive and poor at providing postural stability. The cells also need constant maintenance.

Recline/tilt-in-space - Reclining and tilt-in-space chairs are helpful for pts who lack the ability to do adequate pressure relief otherwise and for pts with orthostatic instability. These chairs are frequently prescribed as backups for pts with power WCs. The addition of these features, however, can significantly increase the size and weight of the WC. Users of reclining WCs may be susceptible to increased spasms and shear forces during the reclining motion. Tilt-in-space WCs offer pressure relief w/o shear and also reduce the likelihood of triggering a spasm during the tilt. Backflow of urine in the tilted position, however, may be an issue in pts with indwelling catheters.

3. Special wheelchairs

"Hemi-chair" - This may be an option for some pts following stroke. The seat height is lowered ~2" and a footrest is removed to allow the neurologically intact foot to propel and steer.

Lower limb amputee - The rear axle is moved posteriorly ~2" to compensate for the rearward displacement of the pt's center of gravity. Turning radius is increased.

One arm drive - This is for unilateral arm amputees or hemiplegics. Both hand rims are on one side. Turning both rims propels the WC; one rim turns the WC. WC width and weight are increased. Good strength and coordination are required.

Standing WC - These chairs have frames that allow the user to passively assume a standing position. The standup position provides pressure relief and weight bearing (which may reduce osteoporosis[1]), and can promote improved bowel/bladder function.

Reference: **1. Goemaere S**: Bone mineral status in paraplegic pts who do or do not perform standing. *Osteoporosis Int* 1994;4:138-43.

B. Electrically Powered Mobility Systems

1. Powered WC

a. **Indications** - This is for pts with physical limitations not compatible with manual wheelchair propulsion (i.e., C1-4, many C5-6 tetraplegics, or severe weakness), and for those with endurance deficits (i.e., severe COPD, cardiac failure) who must conserve their energy for other functions.

b. **User requirements** - Pts must have at least one reproducible movement to access the control system, adequate cognitive and visuoperceptual fxn, proper judgment, and motivation. Ideally, a trial is given to power WC candidates to see if they can eventually learn how to control the WC.

c. **Contraindications** - Failing to meet the user requirements; involuntary motions or inattention that might result in inadvertent activation of the controls.

2. Electric carts (Scooters)

a. **Indications** - It is for pts who can ambulate and transfer but have poor endurance or poor tolerance for prolonged manual WC use secondary to arthropathy or other disease.

b. **User requirements** - Good sitting balance, intact cognitive and visuoperceptual skills, good hand-eye coordination, and adequate function of at least one upper limb to operate the controls are needed.

c. **Caution** - Some models tip over fairly easily, especially at high speeds.

Figures courtesy of **Kottke F**, ed.: *Krusen's Handbook of PM&R*, 4th ed. WB Saunders, 1990.

VIII. Disability

A. WHO Definitions

Impairment - Any loss or abnormality of physiologic, psychological, or anatomic structure or function (e.g., hemiplegia, paraplegia, decreased ROM, pain, BKA, THA, cognitive deficits, depressed mood, aphasia, dysarthria).

Disability (activity limitation) - A restriction, due to an impairment, in the ability to perform an activity w/in the range of what is considered "able-bodied" (e.g., ambulatory/ADL dysfunction, wheelchair use, prone to falls).

Handicap (participation limitation) - A disadvantage resulting from an impairment or disability that limits or prevents the fulfillment of a role that is "normal" for the individual (i.e., unable to care for self, unable to return to previous work/home, unable to participate in leisure activities). Defined by the environment; reflects societal bias.

B. The Americans with Disabilities Act (ADA)

The ADA, passed in 1990, is a federal statute prohibiting discrimination on the basis of disability[1]. **Title I** covers most non-federal employers with ≥15 employees, who must make *reasonable accommodations* in the hiring/maintenance of *qualified disabled persons* (i.e., must be able to do the job's *essential functions*), unless the accommodations pose "undue hardship" on the business. Such accommodations must be *requested* by the applicant/employee; there is no liability for failing to make unrequested provisions. The employer cannot ask applicants about impairments unless they are specifically job-related; pre-employment physicals are allowed only if all applicants are similarly screened. **Titles II and III** cover *access to public facilities** (e.g., parks, doctors' offices, retail stores) and *transportation*. **Title IV** requires that common *telecommunications* carriers provide 24hr services for the hearing and speech impaired (e.g., Telecommunications Device for the Deaf). **Title V** covers miscellaneous provisions.

* To be compliant with ADA guidelines[2], among other things, door widths should have ≥32" clearance when the door is open 90°; hallways and ramps need to be ≥36" wide; ramps should have ≥12" of run for each 1" of rise. The Dept. of Housing & Urban Development's Fair Housing Accessibility Guidelines (1991) cover many of the issues regarding rental apartments.

C. Functional Independence Measure (FIM)[3]

The FIM is widely used to measure the severity of disability and to document the outcomes of rehabilitation. Eighteen items, each scored 1-7 (below), are subgrouped under self-care, sphincter control, locomotion, transfers, communication, and social cognition. (Max score = 18x7 = 126).

No helper	7 Completely independent	(Timely and safely)
	6 Modified independent	(Devices)
Helper (modified dependence)	5 Supervision, setup	(Subject = 100%)
	4 Minimum assist	(Subject = 75%)
	3 Moderate assist	(Subject = 50%)
Helper (complete dependence)	2 Maximum assist	(Subject = 25%)
	1 Total assist	(Dependent)/Not testable

References: **1**. The ADA. Public Law 101-336. **2**. *ADA Accessibility Guidelines for Buildings and Facilities*. U.S. Architectural and Transportation Barriers Board, revised Jan 1998. **3**. *Guide for the Uniform Data Set for Medical Rehabilitation, ver4.0*. SUNY at Buffalo, 1993.

IX. Immobility/ Pressure Ulcers

A. Selected Consequences of Immobility

Muscle atrophy - With complete inactivity, muscle strength is lost at a rate of ~1-3%/day or 10-15%/week, until it plateaus at ~25-40% of the original strength. It takes ~3-5wks for a pt to lose ½ of their muscle strength. This is accompanied by a reduction in muscle size and histologic changes (e.g., ↓ myofibrils/fiber, ↓ fiber cross-sectional area, ↓ # and size of mitochondria). Atrophy occurs faster in certain muscles (quads, hip extensors, and back extensors). As a general rule of thumb, it takes about 2-3× as long to recover muscle strength as it took to lose it.

Soft-tissue contractures - Two-joint muscles are particularly susceptible. Tx of contractures should ideally include sustained terminal stretch (≥20-30mins or more for severe contracture) at least twice a day, ROM exercises, and early mobilization. Stretching can be combined with local heat to the joint (e.g., US). Dynamic splinting, night splints, and serial casting can be options to provide prolonged stretch. Any underlying spasticity should be addressed. CPM may not be very effective in treating fixed contractures because there is no sustained stretch. In selected populations, a surgical intervention such as tenotomy, myotomy, capsulectomy, or soft tissue release may be beneficial.

Cardiovascular and pulmonary - With prolonged bedrest, resting tachycardia (HR increases ~1bpm q2days), inordinate HR responses to submaximal exercise, ↓ stroke volume, ↓ cardiac output, and ↓ VO₂max are noted. Lung function can be compromised with prolonged supine positioning, including decreases in vital capacity, total lung capacity, and functional reserve capacity. Postural hypotension (HR ↑ by ≥20bpm and SBP ↓ ≥20mmHg upon rising) can develop after days to wks of bedrest. Several wks to months may be necessary before cardiovascular postural responses are restored. Tx can include education (gradually changing position before erect sitting or rising), adequate salt and fluid intake, supportive garments (abdominal binders, elastic stockings), use of a tilt-table, and/or medications (β-blockers to reduce tachycardia; ephedrine, phenylephrine, or fludrocortisone to maintain BPs).

Other adverse sequelae - These may include pain, immobilization hypercalcemia or osteoporosis, impaired glucose tolerance, GERD, atelectasis, PE, DVT, bowel/bladder dysfunction, urolithiasis, UTIs, fungal infections, pressure ulcers, peripheral neuropathies, depression, and insomnia, to name a few.

B. Pressure Ulcers

Pressure and shear are direct etiologic factors. Kosiak showed that 70mmHg of pressure applied continuously over 2hrs produced moderate histologic changes in rat muscle[1]. Dinsdale showed that shear can significantly reduce the amount of pressure necessary to disrupt blood flow[2]. 2° factors include immobility, ↓ sensation or mental status, ↑ age, fecal or urinary incontinence (leading to skin maceration), elevated tissue temperatures, circulatory deficiencies, anemia, and nutritional deficits.

Bony prominences are particularly at risk; muscle is more sensitive to breakdown from pressure than skin. Ulcers are commonly staged according to the National Pressure Ulcer Advisory Panel (NPUAP) guidelines:

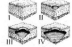

Stage I - Intact epidermis with nonblanchable erythema not resolved w/in 30min. Warmth, edema, induration, or discoloration may be indicators of stage I ulcers in pts with darker skin.

Fig.1, courtesy of NPUAP. *Caveat*: Ulcers with eschars cannot be staged until the eschar is removed.

Stage II - Partial-thickness epidermal or dermal skin loss. These may appear as blisters with erythema.

Stage III - Full-thickness skin loss and subcutaneous involvement, but not through the underlying fascia.

Stage IV - Full-thickness skin loss with involvement of muscle, tendon, bone, or joint.

Pressure ulcer *prevention* should include appropriate seating/ bed equipment, proper positioning, and education about pressure relief (i.e., weight shifting q15-20min for ≥30sec while sitting; turns in bed q2hrs).

Tx of pressure ulcers includes addressing the etiologic factors, tx of infections, debridement of necrotic tissue (sharp, mechanical, enzymatic, or autolytic), regular wound cleansing, and use of appropriate wound dressings **(Fig.2)**. A trial of topical abx (e.g., silver sulfadiazene) may be helpful in wounds not healing with optimal debridement and cleansing. Wound cultures are *not* generally thought to be helpful because most wounds are colonized with bacteria. Systemic abx should be reserved for cases with evidence of osteomyelitis, cellulitis, or systemic infection. Modalities such as UV light, laser radiation, US, hyperbaric O_2, and electrical stimulation may be helpful in accelerating wound repair, although only *E-stim* has sufficient supportive evidence to receive endorsement by the AHCPR (now the AHRQ)[3]. Surgical flaps may expedite the healing of non-infected deep ulcers by filling the void with well-vascularized healthy tissue (they do not provide a "cushion").

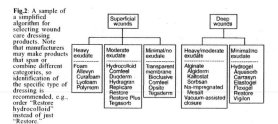

Fig.2: A sample of a simplified algorithm for selecting wound care dressing products. Note that manufacturers may make products that span or combine different categories, so identification of the specific type of dressing is recommended, e.g., order "Restore hydrocolloid" instead of just "Restore."

Superficial wounds			Deep wounds	
Heavy exudate	Moderate exudate	Minimal/no exudate	Heavy/moderate exudate	Minimal/no exudate
Foam Alleyvn Curafoam Lyofoam Polymem	Hydrocolloid Comfeel Duoderm Hydragran Replicare Restore Restore Plus Tegasorb	Transparent membrane Bioclusive Comfeel Opsite Tegaderm	Alginate Algiderm Kaltostat Sorbsan Na-impregnated Mesalt Vacuum-assisted closure	Hydrogel Aquasorb Carrasyn Elastogel Flexigel Restore Vigilon

References: **1. Kosiak M**: Etiology of decubitus ulcers. *Arch PMR* 1961;42:19-29. **2. Dinsdale SN**: Decubitus ulcers: role of presure and friction in causation. *Arch PMR* 1974;55:147-54. **3**. *Clinical Practice Guideline No.3.* AHCPR publication No. 92-0047, 1994. **Fig.2** courtesy of **Priebe M**, University of Texas-Southwestern Medical School/VA North Texas Healthcare System.

X. THERAPEUTIC EXERCISE

A. Muscle Fiber Characteristics

Type I muscle fibers are "slow-twitch," highly fatigue-resistant, grossly dark fibers ("dark meat"), that appear light on myosin ATPase (at pH 9.4) or PAS staining. **Type II** fibers comprise the "white meat" but are dark histologically with these stains. See Table 1 for characteristics of each type/subtype.

All fibers in a given motor unit are of the same type. According to the *Henneman size principle*, smaller motor units are recruited first, then progressively larger units are sequentially recruited as strength of contraction increases.

EMG predominately records type I fiber activity.

FES preferentially recruits type II fibers but may turn IIs into Is after chronic use.

Steroids predominately cause type IIb fiber atrophy. Both types decrease with aging.

	Type I: Slow oxidative (SO)	Type IIA: Fast, oxidative glycolytic (FOG)	Type IIB: Fast glycolytic (FG)
Motor unit type	S	FR	FF
Oxidative capacity	High	Moderately high	Low
Glycolytic capacity	Low	High	Highest
Contractile speed	Slow	Fast	Fast
Fatigue resistance	High	Moderate	Low
Motor unit strength	Low	High	High

FF, fast-fatiguable; FR, fast-fatigue resistant.

Table 1. Characteristics of skeletal muscle fiber subtypes

B. Strength Training

Isometric strengthening - Tension is generated w/o visible joint motion or appreciable change in muscle length (e.g., pushing against a wall). This is most efficient when the exertion occurs at the resting length of the muscle and most useful when joint motion is contraindicated (e.g., s/p tendon repair) or in the setting of pain or inflammation (e.g., RA). Chance of injury is minimized. Isometric exercise should be avoided in the elderly and in pts with HTN due to its tendency to elevate BPs.

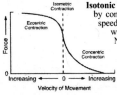

Fig.1 Forces are greatest with high velocity eccentric contractions.

Isotonic strengthening - This is characterized by constant external resistance, but variable speed of movement. Examples include free weights, weight machines (e.g., Nautilus), calisthenics (e.g., pull-ups, push-ups, sit-ups), and TheraBand. The equipment is readily available, but there is potential for injury with this type of exercise.

Isokinetic strengthening - This is characterized by a relatively constant angular joint speed, but variable external resistance. (Special equipment is required, e.g., Cybex, Biodex.) If the user pushes harder, the speed of the manipulated piece of equipment will *not* increase, but the resistance supplied by the machine will. This maximizes resistance throughout the length-tension curve of the exercised muscles and is beneficial in the early phases of rehabilitation. Chance of injury is relatively low.

Fig 2. Acute hemodynamic responses to dynamic (isotonic) vs. isometric exercise

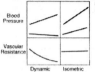

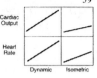

Progressive resistive exercise - In the *DeLorme method*, a 10-repetition maximum (RM) is first determined. Ten reps of the exercise are performed in sets of 50%, 75% and 100% of the 10 RM. The sessions are performed ~3-5×/wk and the 10 RM is redetermined ~qwk. In the *Oxford technique*, the order of the sets is reversed, so that 10reps at 100% of the 10 RM are performed first, followed by sets of 75% and 50%.

The *DeLorme axiom* posits that high-resistance, low-rep exercise builds strength, while low-resistance, high-rep exercise improves endurance[1]. deLateur later demonstrated that for the most part, strength and endurance gains are equivalent for the two types of exercise as long as muscles are exercised to fatigue[2]. High-resistance, low-rep exercise, however, achieves its results more efficiently (fewer reps/less time).

Moritani and deVries demonstrated that gains in the first few wks of strength training were mostly due to neural factors (e.g., improved coordination of muscle firing) and not muscle hypertrophy[3].

C. Aerobic Exercise

Regular aerobic exercise increases VO_2max* and decreases resting BP, whereas strength training does *not* have an effect on either of these. Other long-term cardiovascular adaptations/benefits of aerobic exercise include *increased* stroke volume, cardiac output, work capacity, and HDL; and *decreased* resting HR, HR response to submaximal workloads, and triglyceride levels. Diabetics benefit from reduced obesity and insulin requirements. Improvements in mood, sleep, immune function, and bone density, among others, are also reported in the literature.

Table 2. Example of an aerobic exercise program for a presumably healthy individual[4].

Program phase	Wk #	Exercise dur/ freq (per wk)	Intensity (%VO₂max)	Program phase	Wk #	Exercise dur/ freq (per wk)	Intensity (%VO₂max)
Initial	1	12min/3x	40-50	Improve- ment	6-9	21min/3-4x	70-80
	2	14min/3x	50		10-16	24min/3-4x	70-80
	3	16min/3x	60		17-23	28-30min/4-5x	70-80
	4	18min/3x	60-70		24-27	30min/4-5x	70-85
	5	20min/3x	60-70	Maintenance	28+	30-45min/3x	70-85

*VO_2 is the body's rate of O_2 utilization (mL O_2/kg/min). Once VO_2max is reached, further increases in work rate are powered by anaerobic (glycolytic) metabolism. VO_2max can be calculated by the *Fick equation*: VO_2max = max CO x (a-v O_2 difference), where CO = SV x HR.

References: **1. DeLorme TL:** Restoration of muscle power by heavy-resistance exercises. *JBJS Am* 1945;27:645-67. **2. deLateur BJ:** A test of the DeLorme axiom. *Arch PMR* 1968;49:245-8. **3. Moritani T:** Neural factors vs. hypertrophy in the time course of muscle strength gain. *Am J PMR* 1979;58:115-30. **4.** *ACSM's Guidelines for Exercise Testing and Prescriptions.* Williams & Wilkins, 1995. **Table 1** and figures courtesy of **DeLisa J,** ed.: *Rehabilitation Medicine: Principles and Practice,* 3rd ed. Lippincott-Raven, 1998.

XI. Cardiac Rehabilitation (CR)

A. Introduction

Under the broadened scope of recent AHRQ guidelines, CR may include exercise programs, education and risk factor modification for secondary prevention, and psychosocial counseling[1]. CR is indicated after acute MI, coronary revascularization, cardiac transplantation, or in pts with CHF or chronic stable angina. CR improves VO_2max, peripheral O_2 extraction, ST depression, exercise tolerance, subjective sense of well-being, and return to work rates. It also lowers BP, resting HR, and myocardial O_2 demand. Angiographic studies have showed reduced atherosclerotic lesions in stable angina pts undergoing intensive physical exercise and low-fat diet over 1yr w/o lipid-lowering agents[2]. (It should be noted that it is traditionally stated that CR does *not* raise [improve] anginal threshold, whereas angioplasty and CABG can.)

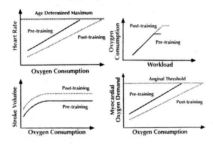

Above: Benefits of CR. Compare pre- (solid lines) vs. post-training (dashed lines).

Figure courtesy of **Braddom R**, ed.: *PM&R*. WB Saunders, 1996

Individual trials of CR after MI have *not* shown a statistically significant lower mortality rate in the CR groups, but a metaanalysis of 22 randomized trials (n=4554) has shown a benefit in overall mortality in the CR group (0.80 odds ratio vs. no CR) during a 3yr avg post-MI period[3].

B. Epidemiology

In 1997, 1.1 million Americans were diagnosed with acute MI, and 800,000 pts underwent coronary revascularization[4]. Limited data suggest that CR is a cost-effective use of medical care resources[1]; however, only 10-20% of appropriate candidates are thought to participate in formal CR programs[4]. Low participation may be due to geographic factors and a failure of physicians to refer pts, particularly the elderly and women.

References: **1. Wenger NK**: Clinical Guideline No.17, AHCPR Publication No.96-0672, 1995 (reviewed by the AHRQ, 2000). **2. Schuler G**: Regular physical exercise and low-fat diet: effects on progression of CAD. Circulation 1992;86:1-11. **3. O'Connor GT**: An overview of randomized trials of rehabilitation with exercise after MI. Circulation 1989;80:234-44. **4. Ades PA**: Cardiac rehabilitation and 2° prevention of coronary heart disease. NEJM 2001;345:892-902.

C. Phases of CR

Phase I - *The inpt training phase* can begin on hospital day 2-4, and typically lasts ~1-2wks. Goals include prevention of the sequelae of immobilization, education and risk factor modification, independent self-care activities, and household distance ambulation on level surfaces. Protocol-limited submaximal stress testing is often done in uncomplicated pts prior to d/c as a guideline for outpatient ADLs and activities.

Phase II - *The outpt training phase* starts 2-4wks post-d/c, and typically lasts 8-12wks. Goals include increasing CV capacity and gradually returning to normal activity levels. A functional exercise tolerance (ECG stress) test is typically done 6-8wks post-cardiac event (which allows time for the formation of a stable scar over the infarcted area) to guide the exercise prescription and determine eligibility for resuming work and sex.

Phase III - *The maintenance phase* is ideally a lifelong program, aimed at maintaining or adding onto benefits obtained during phases I and II, generally under minimal or no clinical supervision.

Absolute contraindications for functional stress testing include recent change on resting ECG or serious cardiac arrhythmias, unstable angina, acute or worsening LV dysfxn, uncontrolled HTN, systemic illness, severe aortic stenosis, or severe physical disability precluding treadmill or arm ergometry use. *Relative contraindications* include hypertrophic cardiomyopathy, electrolyte abnormalities, moderate valvular disease, or significant arterial or pulmonary HTN.

Note: these contraindications for exercise stress testing are similar to the contraindications for CR in general.

D. Exercise prescription

The exercise prescription should address type, intensity, duration and frequency of exercise. *Isotonic, aerobic,* rhythmic exercises involving large muscle groups should be emphasized. Isometrics and resistive exercise are relatively safe in pts with good LV function, but are contraindicated with CHF, severe valvular disease, uncontrolled arrhythmias, or peak exercise capacity <5 METs.

Exercise intensity can be determined by a variety of methods, usually by calculating a "target" HR. The **American Heart Association** method uses 70-85% of the maximum attained by stress testing. For young, healthy adults not undergoing formal exercise stress testing, 70-85% of (220 - age) can also be used for general exercise prescriptions, which is based on the assumption that 220 is the appropriate max for a newborn and that the max decreases ~1bpm/yr. This latter formula, however, does *not* apply after MI.

The **Karvonen formula** calculates a "heart rate zone" which is the resting HR in the sitting position *plus* 40-85% of (max HR determined by exercise tolerance testing minus resting HR). For deconditioned pts, the exercise program should begin at the lower end of the spectrum (i.e., 40-60%) and then increase as fitness improves.

Borg's rating of perceived exertion (RPE) scale is particularly useful for cardiac transplant pts since denervation of the orthotopic heart makes HR parameters unreliable. The traditional Borg RPE scale is scored from 6-20, where 13 is rated as "somewhat hard" and corresponds with an exercise intensity sufficient to provide training benefits but still allow conversation during exercise. 12-13 corresponds to about 60% of max HR; 15 corresponds to 85% of max HR. The Borg scale is probably more psychological than physiological, but encourages independence in exercise (i.e., phase III CR) as external monitoring devices are weaned off.

For pts on β-blockers, training at 85% of symptom-limited HR or 70-90% of the max workload determined by exercise testing is recommended[1]. Pacemakers do not necessarily preclude exercise training in a CR program.

Usual exercise duration/frequency is 20-30min tiw x12wks or more when training at 70% of the max HR. Shorter durations of training on a daily basis for very deconditioned individuals may also be helpful. In general, there is no contraindication to exercising every day, but the likelihood of musculoskeletal injury increases.

E. Post-Cardiac Event Sexual Counseling

Typical criteria for safe resumption of sexual activity after a cardiac event (i.e., MI or CABG) include a stable, asymptomatic pt and tolerance of exercise at 5-7 METs w/o abnormal ECG, BP or HR changes. The time period required is variable but is usually ~6wks post-event for sex with established partners in familiar positions. A useful clinical test is the *two-flight stair-climbing test*: walking for 10mins at 120 paces/min (~3mi/hr or 4.3 METs), then climbing two flights of stairs (~22steps) in 10sec.

Sexual activities associated with sudden death in a cardiac patient include illicit affairs and sex after heavy meals and alcohol intake.

F. Miscellaneous

Sternal precautions - Following sternotomy, typical instructions include no pushing, pulling or lifting objects >5-10lbs for 6-8wks. A "side-rolling" maneuver for getting out of bed is typically taught, and manual wheelchair propulsion is usually prohibited during this time as well.

Cardiac precautions for persons with CAD in non-acute inpt settings - Activity should be terminated if any of the following develops: new onset cardiopulmonary symptoms; HR decreases >20% of baseline; HR increases >50% of baseline; SBP increases to 240mm Hg; SBP decreases ≥30mm Hg from baseline or to <90mm Hg; DBP increases to 120mm Hg[2]. These guidelines were developed by studying 64 physically disabled male pts with CAD using arm ergometers[2]. Individualized parameters for maximum or minimum HR, BP are also frequently used.

New York Heart Association Classification (for CHF and angina)
I. >7 METs tolerated asymptomatically, w/o functional limitation.
II. <6 METs tolerated; but higher levels of activities cause symptoms.
III. Asymptomatic at rest and with most ADLs; >4 METs not tolerated.
IV. Symptomatic at rest and with minimal physical activities.

References: **1. Flores AM, Zohman LR**: Rehab of the cardiac pt. In **DeLisa J**. ed.: *Rehabilitation Medicine: Principles and Practice*, 3rd ed. Lippincott-Raven, 1998. **2. Fletcher BJ**. Cardiac precautions for non-acute inpatient settings. *Am J PMR* 1993;72:140-3.

XII. Pulmonary Rehabilitation (PR)

Rehabilitation for pts with chronic lung conditions is well established and widely accepted as a means of alleviating symptoms and optimizing function[1]. In COPD, PR has been shown to improve dyspnea, exercise capacity, health-related quality of life, and, potentially, survival, while reducing health-care utilization[1]. When considering PR interventions, the respiratory disorders can be generally characterized as *ventilatory disorders* (CO_2 retention) or *obstructive disorders* (oxygen impairment)[2].

Ventilatory disorders (restrictive or mechanical disorders) - These can be caused by neuromuscular or skeletal disorders that decrease respiratory muscle function (e.g., myopathy, motor neuron disease, myelopathy, MS, chest wall deformity). Keys to clinical monitoring include spirometry for VC and max insufflation capacity, peak cough flows, and non-invasive CO_2 monitoring. Expiratory flow should exceed 160L/min (~3L/sec) for secretions to be adequately cleared from the airways[2]. If these flows cannot be achieved naturally, insufflation followed by a caregiver-provided abdominal thrust ("quad cough") or use of an *insufflator-exsufflator device* (CoughAssist, Respironics) may be beneficial. Invasive suctioning is a less ideal alternative. *Glossopharyngeal breathing* can be used to maximize insufflation and can serve as a back-up in the event of ventilator failure[2].

Respiratory muscles can be aided by devices such as mouthpiece or nasal intermittent positive pressure ventilators (*IPPV*) and intermittent abdominal-pressure ventilators (*IAPV*)[2]. The latter can augment TV by 250-1200mL[2]. CPAP and BiPAP can be useful at night in pts with obstructive sleep apnea by keeping airways patent. Intubation, tracheostomy, and supplemental oxygen therapy are probably overutilized in pts with ventilatory disorders, whereas non-invasive assisted ventilation and assisted cough are probably underutilized.

Obstructive disorders (intrinsic disorders) - These include COPD, asthmatic bronchitis, and cystic fibrosis. Medical management may include inhalers and/or nebulizers. *Lower limb exercise and ambulation programs* can greatly improve exercise tolerance and are strongly recommended for pts with COPD[1]. Inspiratory resistance training (ventilatory muscle training) may be helpful in select, highly motivated populations of COPD pts who remain symptomatic despite optimal therapy[1]. *Pursed-lip breathing* (slow exhaling through pursed lips to reduce small airway collapse) can help manage dyspnea. Long-term psychological interventions, e.g., relaxation therapy, have yet to be proven beneficial in randomized controlled trials, but are supported by expert opinion[1].

Supplemental home O_2 may be indicated when pO_2 is consistently ≤55-60mm Hg. Medicare guidelines[3] for coverage of home O_2 generally require documentation of resting, sleep, or exercise pO_2 ≤55mm Hg or SaO_2 ≤88% (on room air). Pts with pO_2s of 56-59% or a SaO_2 of 89% may be eligible with concomitant CHF, pulmonary HTN, or other criteria.

References: **1.** Ries AL: Pulmonary rehabilitation: Joint American College of Chest Physicians/American Association of Cardiovascular and Pulmonary Rehabilitation evidence-based guidelines. *Chest* 1997;112:1363-96. **2.** Bach JR: Pulmonary rehabilitation. In **O'Young BJ**, ed.: *PMR Secrets*, 2nd ed. Hanley & Belfus, 2002. **3.** Medicare carriers manual, claim processing, Part 3. HCFA Publication 14-3: PB94-954799, 1994.

XIII. Rheumatology

A. Hip and Knee Osteoarthritis (OA)

OA, the most prevalent form of arthritis in the U.S., is due to a disruption of the normal process of degradation and synthesis of articular cartilage and subchondral bone[1]. Biomechanical and biologic factors are implicated. Age and obesity are among the risk factors; joint involvement is typically asymmetric. Weight-bearing joints are usually involved.

American College of Rheumatology (ACR) criteria[2] for dx of *hip OA* include hip pain and 2 of the following: ESR<20, femoral or acetabular osteophytes, or joint space narrowing. ACR criteria for *knee OA* include knee pain and osteophytes and $\geq$1 of the following: age >50yrs, morning joint stiffness $\leq$30min duration, or crepitus on motion.

1. Non-pharmacologic management

Strengthening and aerobic exercises (e.g., fitness walking) have been shown in numerous trials to reduce pain and disability while improving quality of life. The Fitness Arthritis and Seniors Trial (FAST) confirmed the beneficial effects of *quadriceps strengthening* and aerobic exercise in pts with knee OA[3]. Felsen reported that a decrease of 2 body mass index units (~11.2lbs) over 10yrs in a group of women above median BMI decreased the odds of developing OA by over 50%[4].

To promote self-management and improve compliance, pts should be encouraged to participate in programs such as the *Arthritis Foundation Self-Help Course*. For pts who are poorly tolerant of weight-bearing exercises due to their OA, *aquatic exercises* may be an alternative. (Swimming, however, may worsen lumbar facet arthritis symptoms.) *Physical modalities* and *judicious rest* between sessions may also improve tolerance and compliance with exercises.

A *cane* held in the hand contralateral to a painful hip can help unload the joint (see p.30) and make ambulation more bearable. For a painful knee, the cane can be held in either hand[5]. *Knee unloading braces* and *lateral heel wedges* can reduce stress in the medial knee compartment and relieve pain. *Environmental adaptations* include raising toilet and chair heights.

2. Pharmacologic options, per ACR

Pharmaceutical agents are most effective when combined with non-pharmacologic strategies[6]. A trial of *acetaminophen* is recommended as the initial tx for mild-moderate hip OA or knee OA w/o gross inflammation due to its overall cost, efficacy, and toxicity profile[6]. For pts with moderate-severe knee OA and signs of joint inflammation, *intraarticular (IA) steroids*, *COX-2 inhibitors*, or *NSAIDs* (with misoprostol or a proton pump inhibitor if the pt is at risk for adverse upper GI events) may be considered as first line therapy[6].

Tramadol can be considered in pts with moderate-severe pain with contraindications to NSAIDs/COX-2 and/or failing other txs. The mean effective dose for tramadol has generally been ~200-300mg, divided in 4 doses[6]. More potent opioids can be considered for pts not tolerating or failing tramadol.

Topical analgesics (e.g., methylsalicylate or capsaicin) can be considered in pts with mild-moderate knee OA pain as an adjunctive tx or as monotherapy. *IA hyaluronan* therapy (e.g., Synvisc) is indicated for pts with knee (*not* hip) OA with a poor response to simple analgesics and nonpharmacologic tx. Studies of IA hyaluronan are somewhat controversial and inconclusive, but generally seem to favor its use in mild-moderate knee OA[6]. Peak effects may be at 8-12wks; duration of action may be up to 6mos. Limited data are available regarding the efficacy of multiple courses of IA hyaluronan. *IA glucocorticoids* fluoroscopically guided into the hip joint may be efficacious in some pts[6].

3. Alternative and investigational txs

Complementary and alternative medicine txs abound. Studies of *glucosamine/chondroitin* appear promising at providing modest short-term symptomatic improvement. Much of the published research to date, however, is qualitatively suboptimal. A major ($14million) NIH-sponsored multi-center trial is expected to be completed in 2005. Research on the efficacy of *acupuncture* in OA is likewise promising but qualitatively suboptimal. Other txs under ongoing investigation include supplementation with *vitamin D* and the *antioxidant vitamins* A, C, E, and coenzyme Q10.

A recent development in the surgical tx of knee OA is the *UniSpacer*, which is FDA-approved for isolated, moderate, medial compartment OA. The kidney-bean shaped lightweight metallic-alloy device is a self-centering bearing that requires no shaving of bone or screw/cement fixation to the native anatomy. Long-term efficacy is under investigation.

References: 1. **Klippel J**, ed.: *Primer on the Rheumatic Diseases*, 12th ed. Arthritis Foundation, 2001. 2. **Hochberg MC**: Guideline for the medical management of OA. *Arthritis Rheum* 1995;38:1535-46. 3. **Ettinger WH**: A randomized trial comparing aerobic exercise and resistance exercise with a health education program in older adults with knee OA [FAST]. *JAMA* 1997;277:25-31. 4. **Felsen DT**: Weight loss reduces the risk for symptomatic knee OA in women. The Framingham Study. *Ann Intern Med* 1992;116:589-9. 5. **Vargo MM**: Contralateral vs. ipsilateral cane use. Effects on muscles crossing the knee joint. *Am J PMR* 1992;71:170-6. 6. **ACR guidelines**: Recommendations for the medical management of OA of the hip and knee: 2000 update. *Arthritis Rheum* 2000;43:1905-15.

B. Rheumatoid Arthritis (RA)

RA is a chronic systemic inflammatory disorder affecting women > men with ~1% prevalence in the U.S. RA can cause an erosive, polyarticular, typically symmetric synovitis and extraarticular manifestations, such as fatigue, anemia, rheumatoid nodules, cardiac valve abnormalities, and pericarditis. Classic physical exam findings include boutonniere's, swan neck, or mallet finger deformities, symmetric wrist swelling, Baker's cysts, MCP subluxation with ulnar deviation of the fingers, and DIP joint sparing.

ACR criteria for the dx of RA[1] are (≥4 of the following 7 items) morning stiffness ≥1hr*, soft-tissue swelling/fluid around ≥3 joint areas*, ≥1 joint area involvement in the hand/wrist*, simultaneous symmetric joint area involvement*, rheumatoid nodules, +serum RF, and X-ray changes (PA hand/wrist films demonstrating marginal erosions or juxtaarticular osteopenia of the involved joints).

*For at least 6wks. Reference: 1. **Arnett FC**: The American Rheumatism Association 1987 revised criteria for the classification of RA. *Arthritis Rheum* 1988;31:315-24.

1. RA management

ROM exercises and *stretching* should be regularly practiced. *Isometric* strengthening exercises are preferred to minimize joint inflammation. *Splints*, particularly resting wrist-hand splints and knee or hindfoot splints, are helpful in reducing pain and preventing progression of deformity. A dorsal hand orthosis with an ulnar aspect MCP block and individual finger stops can be useful in the setting of ulnar deviation. Education should emphasis *avoidance of overuse* and *joint protection techniques* (e.g., decreasing activity during flare-ups, modifying activities to reduce joint stress, using splints, and maintaining strength).

NSAIDs or *COX-2* inhibitors alone may be helpful symptomatically in mild or early disease. Pts with high titers of RF, extra-articular involvement, or more severe disease may be candidates for *disease-modifying antirheumatic drugs* (DMARDs), which offer symptomatic relief and also have been shown to modify disease progression. Examples include methotrexate, leflunomide, cyclosporine, sulfasalazine, parenteral gold, and hydroxy-chloroquine. Due to their significant side effects, long-term steroids are reserved for pts unresponsive to other txs.

Newer agents (recently FDA-approved) known as *biological response modifiers* (BRMs) also improve symptoms and modify disease progression, but have fewer of the non-specific side effects that often complicate tx with traditional DMARDs. Examples include the IL-1 inhibitor *anakinra* (Kineret) and TNF-α inhibitors *etanercept* (Enbrel) and *infliximab* (Remicade). Recent trends have been to initiate tx with DMARDs or BRMs earlier and to use agents in combination (i.e., methotrexate plus a 2nd agent have been shown to virtually halt radiographic progression of RA over 2yrs[1]).

Arthroscopic *synovectomy* can be performed to reduce joint destruction and relieve symptoms not alleviated by conservative management.

2. Juvenile rheumatoid arthritis (JRA)[2,3]

JRA is the most common childhood chronic arthritis, affecting some 70,000-100,000 persons <16yrs of age in the U.S. Girls are more frequently affected than boys, although this may vary with JRA subtype. Dx requires onset prior to age 16yrs, persistent arthritis in ≥1 joints for ≥6wks, and exclusion of other childhood arthritides. RF is usually negative. Subtypes include *systemic-onset JRA* (Still's disease; 10% of cases, variable # of joints affected), *polyarticular JRA* (40% of cases, ≥5 joints), and *pauciarticular JRA* (50% of cases, ≤4 joints). ANA-seropositive girls of the pauciarticular subtype are at particular risk for *uveitis*, which can lead to blindness. >30% of JRA patients have significant functional limitations after ≥10yrs of f/u. Many children do not reach the expected adult height. Mortality rates are 3-14× greater than expected.

Tx: NSAIDs, methotrexate, and intraarticular steroids (i.e., for acutely inflamed joints) can be used for pain control. *Prone lying* and *splints* may prevent/correct contractures. *Heat* for non-acutely inflamed joints may help reduce stiffness. Swimming, cycling, and isometric exercises are relatively less stressful to the joints.

References: 1. Kremer JM: Rational use of new and existing DMARDs in RA. *Ann Intern Med* 2001;134:695-706. 2. Klippel J, ed.: *Primer on the Rheumatic Diseases*, 12th ed. Arthritis Foundation, 2001. 3. Molnar G, ed.: *Pediatric Rehabilitation*, 3rd ed. Hanley & Belfus, 1999.

C. Ankylosing Spondylitis (AS)

AS is one of the spondyloarthropathies. ♂:♀ is 3:1; onset is typically in late adolescence or early adulthood; 90% are HLA-B27 positive[1]. Initial symptoms include pain and stiffness in the buttock or lumbar area, which are worse with inactivity and improve with exercise or hot showers. B/l, symmetric *sacroiliitis* is a characteristic early X-ray finding. Inflammation of the spine can lead to *syndesmophyte* formation, then ultimately to a kyphotic bony ankylosis ("*bamboo spine*"). Progression of spinal inflexibility can be followed by *Schober's test*. Although the course of AS is variable, the majority of pts have mild disease and normal longevity[1]. Extraarticular manifestations usually affect the eye. *Uveitis* may present as acute monocular pain and photophobia progressing to blindness.

Tx includes *spinal extension exercises* (e.g., swimming, push-ups), expansive chest breathing, pectoral and hip flexor stretching, and prone lying. A *hard mattress*, preferably w/o pillows behind the head, should be recommended. NSAIDs (e.g., naproxen, indomethacin) may reduce pain and symptoms of spinal stiffness. Recently, *etanercept*, a TNF-α inhibitor, was shown to improve quality of life, function, and pain/stiffness in a small randomized, double-masked, placebo-controlled trial[2].

References: **1.** Klippel J, ed.: *Primer on the Rheumatic Diseases,* 12th ed. Arthritis Foundation, 2001. **2. Gorman JD**: Treatment of AS by inhibition of TNF-α. *NEJM* 2002;246:1349-56.

D. Fibromyalgia (FM)

FM is an incompletely understood clinical syndrome affecting women much more frequently than men. It is characterized by widespread, chronic pain and systemic symptoms (e.g., fatigue, sleep disturbance, depression).

American College of Rheumatology criteria[1] include 1) **pain and tenderness lasting for ≥3mos** (involving bilateral sides, plus above and below the waist; in addition, axial skeletal pain must be present) *and* 2) **pain in 11 or more of 18 predetermined tender points on exam** (see below right), elicited by applying approximately 4kg/cm pressure (enough to blanche a fingernail).

Tx should include *education* (e.g., FM typically has a non-progressive course), low-impact *aerobic activities*, and analgesia. Pharmaceutical options include low dose *tricyclic antidepressants* at bedtime, *SSRIs, NSAIDs,* tramadol, and tender point injections. TENS, acupuncture, massage, and relaxation therapy are other options. Underlying depression should be addressed.

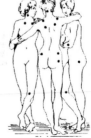

Right: *FM tender point test areas:* 1. suboccipital muscle insertions; 2. low anterior cervical; 3. second costochondral junction; 4. upper border trapezius; 5. supraspinatus; 6. distal lateral epicondyle area; 7. superior-lateral gluteal area; 8. posterior to greater trochanter; 9. medial knee.

Reference: **1. Wolfe F**: The ACR 1990 criteria for the classification of fibromyalgia. *Arthritis Rheum* 1990;33:160-72. Figure copyrighted 1990 by John Wiley & Sons, Inc. Reprinted with permission of Wiley-Liss, Inc., a subsidiary of John Wiley & Sons, Inc.

XIV. PERIPHERAL NERVOUS SYSTEM
A. Dermatomes

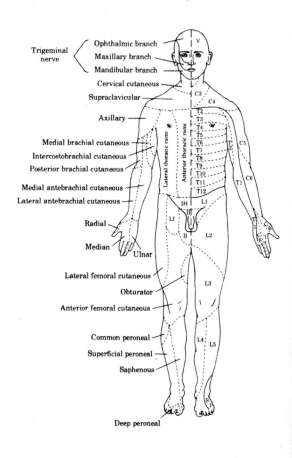

Trigeminal nerve
— Ophthalmic branch
— Maxillary branch
— Mandibular branch
— Cervical cutaneous
Supraclavicular
Axillary
Medial brachial cutaneous
Intercostobrachial cutaneous
Posterior brachial cutaneous
Medial antebrachial cutaneous
Lateral antebrachial cutaneous
Radial
Median
Ulnar
Lateral femoral cutaneous
Obturator
Anterior femoral cutaneous
Common peroneal
Superficial peroneal
Saphenous
Deep peroneal

Lateral thoracic rami
Anterior thoracic rami

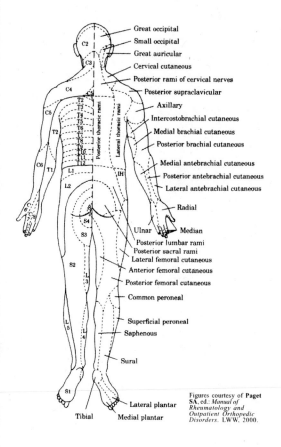

Great occipital
Small occipital
Great auricular
Cervical cutaneous
Posterior rami of cervical nerves
Posterior supraclavicular
Axillary
Intercostobrachial cutaneous
Medial brachial cutaneous
Posterior brachial cutaneous
Medial antebrachial cutaneous
Posterior antebrachial cutaneous
Lateral antebrachial cutaneous
Radial
Ulnar   Median
Posterior lumbar rami
Posterior sacral rami
Lateral femoral cutaneous
Anterior femoral cutaneous
Posterior femoral cutaneous
Common peroneal
Superficial peroneal
Saphenous
Sural
Lateral plantar
Tibial   Medial plantar

Figures courtesy of **Paget SA**, ed.: *Manual of Rheumatology and Outpatient Orthopedic Disorders.* LWW, 2000.

B. Brachial Plexus

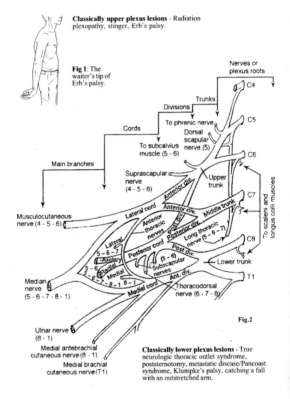

Classically upper plexus lesions - Radiation plexopathy, stinger, Erb's palsy.

Fig 1: The waiter's tip of Erb's palsy.

Nerves or plexus roots

Trunks

Divisions

Cords

To phrenic nerve

Dorsal scapular nerve (5)

To subcalvius muscle (5 - 6)

Main branches

Suprascapular nerve (4 - 5 - 6)

Anterior div.

Lateral cord

Anterior div.

Anterior thoracic nerves

Musculocutaneous nerve (4 - 5 - 6)

Lateral

5 - 6 - 7

Axillary 5 - 6

Radial

Medial 5 - 6 - 7 - 8 - 1

Posterior cord

Post div.

Subscapular nerves (5 - 6)

Median nerve (5 - 6 - 7 - 8 - 1)

Medial cord

Ant. div.

Thoracodorsal nerve (6 - 7 - 8)

Ulnar nerve (8 - 1)

Medial antebrachial cutaneous nerve (8 - 1)

Medial brachial cutaneous nerve (T1)

Upper trunk

Middle trunk

Long thoracic nerve (5 - 6 - 7)

Lower trunk

To scaleni and longus colli muscles

C4

C5

C6

C7

C8

T1

Fig.2

Classically lower plexus lesions - True neurologic thoracic outlet syndrome, poststernotomy, metastatic disease/Pancoast syndrome, Klumpke's palsy, catching a fall with an outstretched arm.

Fig.2 courtesy of **Waxman S**. ed.: *Correlative Neuroanatomy*. 22nd ed. Appleton & Lange, 1995.

C. Peripheral Motor Innervation

1. Median nerve

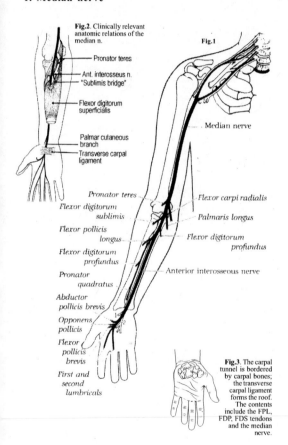

Fig.2. Clinically relevant anatomic relations of the median n.

- Pronator teres
- Ant. interosseus n.
- "Sublimis bridge"
- Flexor digitorum superficialis
- Palmar cutaneous branch
- Transverse carpal ligament

Fig.1

Median nerve

Pronator teres
Flexor digitorum sublimis
Flexor pollicis longus
Flexor digitorum profundus
Pronator quadratus
Abductor pollicis brevis
Opponens pollicis
Flexor pollicis brevis
First and second lumbricals

Flexor carpi radialis
Palmaris longus
Flexor digitorum profundus
Anterior interosseous nerve

Fig.3. The carpal tunnel is bordered by carpal bones; the transverse carpal ligament forms the roof. The contents include the FPL, FDP, FDS tendons and the median nerve.

Fig.1 courtesy of **Dawson DM**, ed.: *Entrapment Neuropathies*, 3rd ed. Lippincott-Raven, 1999. **Fig.2** courtesy of **Stewart JD**: *Focal Peripheral Neuropathies*, 3rd ed. LWW, 2000.

2. Ulnar nerve

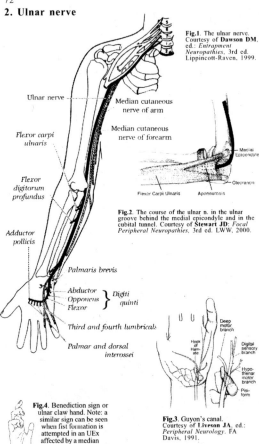

Ulnar nerve

Median cutaneous
nerve of arm

Median cutaneous
nerve of forearm

Flexor carpi
ulnaris

Flexor
digitorum
profundus

Adductor
pollicis

Palmaris brevis

Abductor
Opponens } Digiti
Flexor   quinti

Third and fourth lumbricals

Palmar and dorsal
interossei

Fig.1. The ulnar nerve. Courtesy of **Dawson DM**, ed.: *Entrapment Neuropathies*, 3rd ed. Lippincott-Raven, 1999.

Medial Epicondyle

Olecranon

Flexor Carpi Ulnaris   Aponeurosis

Fig.2. The course of the ulnar n. in the ulnar groove behind the medial epicondyle and in the cubital tunnel. Courtesy of **Stewart JD**: *Focal Peripheral Neuropathies*, 3rd ed. LWW, 2000.

Deep motor branch

Hook of Hamate

Digital sensory branch

Hypothenar motor branch

Pisiform

Fig.3. Guyon's canal. Courtesy of **Liveson JA**, ed.: *Peripheral Neurology*. FA Davis, 1991.

Fig.4. Benediction sign or ulnar claw hand. Note: a similar sign can be seen when fist formation is attempted in an UEx affected by a median neuropathy. Courtesy of **Magee D**: *Orthopedic Physical Assessment*, 3rd ed. WB Saunders, 1997.

Fig.5. Froment's sign is substitution of the FPL for a weak adductor pollicus when a pt is asked to hold a piece of paper in the first web space. Courtesy of **Magee D**: *Orthopedic Physical Assessment*, 3rd ed: WB Saunders, 1997.

3. Axillary and radial nerves

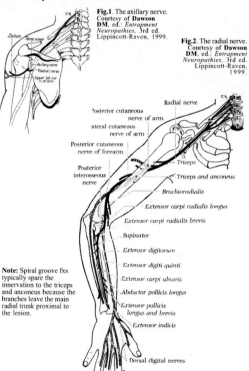

Fig.1. The axillary nerve. Courtesy of **Dawson DM**, ed.: *Entrapment Neuropathies*, 3rd ed. Lippincott-Raven, 1999.

Deltoid
Teres minor
Axillary nerve
Radial nerve
Upper lat cut n of arm

Fig.2. The radial nerve. Courtesy of **Dawson DM**, ed.: *Entrapment Neuropathies*, 3rd ed. Lippincott-Raven, 1999.

Radial nerve

Posterior cutaneous nerve of arm

ateral cutaneous nerve of arm

Posterior cutaneous nerve of forearm

Posterior interosseous nerve

Triceps

Triceps and anconeus

Brachioradialis

Extensor carpi radialis longus

Extensor carpi radialis brevis

Supinator

Extensor digitorum

Extensor digiti quinti

Extensor carpi ulnaris

Abductor pollicis longus

Extensor pollicis longus and brevis

Extensor indicis

Dorsal digital nerves

Note: Spiral groove fxs typically spare the innervation to the triceps and anconeus because the branches leave the main radial trunk proximal to the lesion.

Fig.3. Monteggia's fx (fx of ulnar diaphysis with radial head dislocation) can cause a posterior interosseous n. lesion. Courtesy of **Hoppenfeld S**: *Treatment & Rehabilitation of Fxs.* LWW, 2000.

Fig.4. Galeazzi's fx (distal radius fx with disruption of the distal radioulnar articulation) is also known to cause posterior interosseous n. lesions.

4. LEx nerves

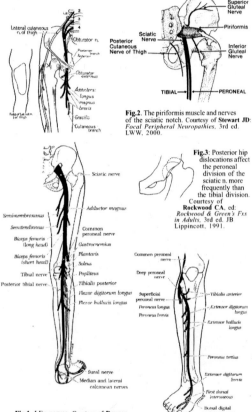

Lateral cutaneous n. of thigh

2
3
4

Obturator n.

Posterior branch
Anterior

Obturator externus

Adductors:
longus
magnus
brevis

Gracilis

Cutaneous branch

Ridge of patella (or thigh)

Fig.2. The piriformis muscle and nerves of the sciatic notch. Courtesy of **Stewart JD**: *Focal Peripheral Neuropathies,* 3rd ed. LWW, 2000.

Superior Gluteal Nerve

Piriformis

Sciatic Nerve

Posterior Cutaneous Nerve of Thigh

Inferior Gluteal Nerve

TIBIAL — PERONEAL

Fig.3: Posterior hip dislocations affect the peroneal division of the sciatic n. more frequently than the tibial division. Courtesy of **Rockwood CA**, ed: *Rockwood & Green's Fxs in Adults,* 3rd ed. JB Lippincott, 1991.

Sciatic nerve

Semimembranosus

Semitendinosus

Biceps femoris (long head)

Biceps femoris (short head)

Tibial nerve

Posterior tibial nerve

Adductor magnus

Common peroneal nerve

Gastrocnemius

Plantaris

Soleus

Popliteus

Tibialis posterior

Flexor digitorum longus

Flexor hallucis longus

Sural nerve

Median and lateral calcanean nerves

Common peroneal nerve

Deep peroneal nerve

Superficial peroneal nerve

Peroneus longus

Peroneus brevis

Tibialis anterior

Extensor digitorum longus

Extensor hallucis longus

Peroneus tertius

Extensor digitorum brevis

First dorsal interosseous

Dorsal digital cutaneous nerve

Fig.1. LEx nerves. Courtesy of **Dawson DM**, ed.: *Entrapment Neuropathies,* 3rd ed. Lippincott-Raven, 1999.

D. Classification of peripheral nerves

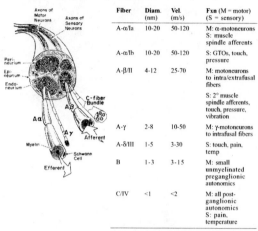

Fiber	Diam. (nm)	Vel. (m/s)	Fxn (M = motor) (S = sensory)
A-α/Ia	10-20	50-120	M: α-motoneurons S: muscle spindle afferents
A-α/Ib	10-20	50-120	S: GTOs, touch, pressure
A-β/II	4-12	25-70	M: motoneurons to intra/extrafusal fibers S: 2° muscle spindle afferents, touch, pressure, vibration
A-γ	2-8	10-50	M: γ-motoneurons to intrafusal fibers
A-δ/III	1-5	3-30	S: touch, pain, temp
B	1-3	3-15	M: small unmyelinated preganglionic autonomics
C/IV	<1	<2	M: all post-ganglionic autonomics S: pain, temperature

Reference: **I. Dumitru D**: *Electrodiagnostic Medicine*, 2nd ed. Hanley & Belfus, 2002. **Figure** courtesy of **Cousins M**, ed.: *Neural Blockade in Clinical Anesthesia and Management of Pain*, 3rd ed. Lippincott-Raven, 1998.

Supplement: A dDx of Weakness

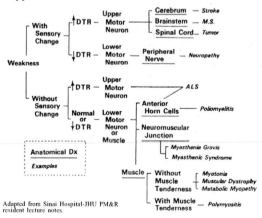

Adapted from Sinai Hospital-JHU PM&R resident lecture notes.

XV. Electrodiagnostics (EDx)

A. Nerve Conduction Studies (NCS)

1. Selected *sample* EDx laboratory normal values

NCS	Stim	Rec	Dist (cm)	Amp	Lat(ms)	Original reference
SENSORY				*pk-pk*	*pk*	
median	mid-palm	index	7	------	2.2	Felsenthal
median	wrist	index	14	10μV	3.7	Melvin/Felsenthal
median	wrist	middle	14	9μV	3.7	Melvin
ulnar	wrist	little	14	10μV	3.7	Johnson
(median/ulnar latency difference should be <0.5ms)						Felsenthal
ulnar DC	forearm	dors hand	8	8μV	2.6	Jabre
radial	forearm	EPL	14	13μV	3.3	MacKenzie/DeLisa
radial	forearm	1st web	10	10μV	2.7	Cleveland Clinic
sural	calf	lat mall	14	5μV	4.4	Izzo
sup per	lat calf	ankle	10	6μV	3.2	DiBenedetto
sup per	lat calf	lat mall	12	8μV	3.6	Jabre
MIXED						
median	palm	wrist	8	40μV	2.3	Med Coll Georgia
ulnar	palm	wrist	8	11μV	2.2	Med Coll Georgia
(median/ulnar latency difference should be <0.5ms)						Redmond/MCG
tibial	med plant	ankle	14	11μV	3.7	DeLisa
tibial	lat plant	ankle	14	9μV	3.7	DeLisa
(lat plant SNAP absence after age 55 not significant)						Mayo Clinic
MOTOR				*on-pk*	*on*	
median	wrist	APB	8	5.0mV	4.3	Melvin
(median/ulnar latency difference should be <1.2ms)						Felsenthal
ulnar	wrist	ADM	8	2.5mV	4.2	Melvin/Checkles
(difference to FDI should be <2ms)						Olney
ulnar	SSIS	ADM	1	------	0.4	Campbell
tibial	med mall	AH	10	3.5mV	5.4	Oh
tibial	med mall	ADQP	12	3.0mV	6.2	Oh
peroneal	ankle	EDB	8	2.6mV	6.2	Ma

NCS VELOCITY

UEx	48-70 m/s
LEx	39-55 m/s
(≥10 m/s drop in CV across 2 points is significant)	Payan/Eisen

The above is an unpublished compilation of EDx normal values used by resident physicians at the Sinai Hospital of Baltimore-Johns Hopkins University PM&R training program on some of their EDx rotations. This table is presented as *one* example of a set of reference values. In practice, each EDx laboratory should establish its own reference values. This compilation was originally prepared by N.Spellman, T.Dillingham, et al. for Walter Reed AMC. Space limitations preclude a full listing of the original references cited above.

2. Effects of temperature and age on NCS[1]

Cooling is thought to prolong the opening of Na+ channels. As temperatures ↓, amplitudes and latencies of SNAPs and CMAPs ↑. Henrickson reported a 2.4m/s per degree change w/in the range of 29-38°C for human UEx motor NCVs[2]. Correction formulae for low temperatures exist, but their use is discouraged. The best approach is to warm a cool limb prior to the NCS (UEx: 32°C; LEx: 30°C).

In the elderly, SNAP and CMAP amplitudes are decreased and latencies are increased. Motor NCVs are about 50% of adult values at birth. Normal adult values are attained by age 3-5 yrs. After age 50yrs, there is a progressive decline of ~1-2m/s per decade in the NCVs of the fastest motor fibers.

3. Filter effects on NCS[1]

Sequential elevation of the **LOW FREQ** (high pass) filter (A-D) decreases peak latency and amplitude of **SNAP**s.

Trace	Low frequency	Latency Onset	Latency Peak	Duration negative spike	Amplitude
	Hz	ms	ms	ms	μv
A	1	2.6	3.3	1.4	65
B	10	2.6	3.3	1.4	65
C	100	2.6	3.1	1.0	54
D	300	2.6	3.0	0.8	30

Reducing the **HIGH FREQ** (low pass) filter (A-D) increases onset and peak latency and slightly decreases the amplitude of **SNAP**s.

Trace	High frequency filter	Latency Onset	Latency Peak	Amplitude
	Hz	ms	ms	μV
A	10,000	2.7	3.3	76
B	2,000	2.8	3.4	76
C	1,000	2.8	3.8	75
D	500	3.0	4.2	64

Sequential elevation of the **LOW FREQ** (high pass) filter (A-C) decreases peak latency and amplitude of **CMAP**s.

Trace	Low frequency filter	Latency Onset	Latency Peak	Amplitude
	Hz	ms	ms	mV
A	1	3.5	6.7	21
B	10	3.5	6.3	21
C	100	3.5	5.0	11

Reducing the **HIGH FREQ** (low pass) filter (A-D) increases onset and peak latency, but may not affect the amplitude of **CMAP**s.

Trace	High frequency filter	Latency Onset	Latency Peak	Amplitude
	Hz	ms	ms	mV
A	10,000	3.3	6.9	21
B	2,000	3.5	7.1	21
C	1,000	3.8	7.3	21
D	500	4.2	7.5	21

References: **1. Dumitru D**, ed.: *EDx Medicine*, 2nd ed. Hanley & Belfus, 2002. **2. Henrickson JD**: Conduction velocity of motor nerves in normal subjects and patients with neuromuscular disorders. [Thesis] University of Minnesota, 1956. In: **Dumitru D**, ed.: *EDx Medicine*, 2nd ed. Hanley & Belfus, 2002. Filter effects figures courtesy of **Dumitru D**: Practical instrumentation and common sources of error. *Am J PMR* 1988;67:55-65.

78
4. Late Responses[1]

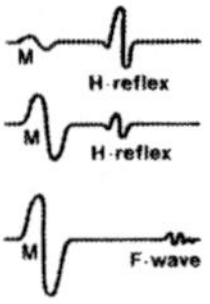

The *H (Hoffmann) reflex* is a CMAP elicited by submaximal stimulation of the afferent limb of a monosynaptic reflex arc. It disappears with supramaximal stimuli. It is typically used to assess S1 radiculopathy (tibial n./gastroc-soleus), and sometimes to study the C6,7 roots (median n./FCR).

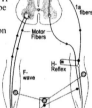

Fig.1

A mean tibial H-reflex of 29.8±2.74ms has been reported. Predicted latencies increase with limb length and age, and can be estimated using a standard nomogram (not pictured). The side-to-side difference should be <1.5ms for the tibial H reflex (<1.8 for ages 60-88). The H-reflex may be absent in the elderly.

The *F (foot) wave* is an antidromic motoneuron volley, *not* a reflex, and is used to assess proximal nerve conduction (but *not* radiculopathy). It can be obtained from most muscles by a supramaximal stimulus. Reference values are listed below. The side-to-side difference should be <2ms for UEx responses, and <4ms for the LEx responses.

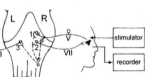

median F (wrist)	29.1 ±2.3ms
ulnar F (wrist)	30.5 ±3.0ms
peroneal F (ankle)	51.3 ±4.7ms
tibial F (ankle)	52.3 ±4.3ms

Fig.2

The *blink reflex* is used to assess the supraorbital n. (CN V, afferent), facial n. to the orbicularis oculi (CN VII, efferent), and selected brainstem areas, as diagrammed in the proposed pathway (see Fig.3).

The "R1" response is produced by the ipsilateral CN V-CN VII reflex arc (#1 on Fig.3). A caudal pathway synapses with the b/l facial nuclei to produce the ipsilateral and contralateral "R2" responses (#2,3 on Fig.3). Reference values (ms) are listed below:

Fig.3

stim	record	R1	R2(ipsi)	R2(contra)
supraorb	orb ocu	<13.1	<41.0	<43.0

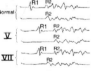

A CN V lesion delays the R1 and b/l R2 responses. An *ipsilateral* CN VII lesion delays the R1 and ipsilateral R2, while the contralateral R2 is normal. A *contralateral* CN VII lesion (not pictured) delays the contralateral R2 only.

Fig.4

References: 1. **Dumitru D**, ed.: *Electrodiagnostic Medicine*, 2nd ed. Hanley & Belfus, 2002. **Figs.1,2** courtesy of **Oh SJ**: *Principles of Clinical Electromyography: Case Studies*, LWW, 1998. **Figs.3,4** from **Kimura J**: *Electrodiagnosis in Diseases of Nerve and Muscle*, 2nd ed. Copyrighted by Oxford University Press, Inc., 1989, modified with permission.

B. EMG

1. Monopolar vs. concentric needles[1]

Monopolar needles produce CMAPs with larger amplitudes and but essentially the same durations as concentric needles. Removing the teflon from a monopolar needle will diminish CMAP amplitude.

Concentric needles will produce fewer polyphasics and less distant activity (less electrical noise), but may have a decreased sensitivity for recording spontaneous activity. Generally, concentric needles are more expensive and less well-tolerated by patients, although newer, smaller gauge (26-g, 27-g) needles are now available and are well-tolerated. Unlike the monopolar needle, there is *no* need for a separate reference electrode.

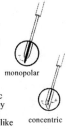

monopolar

concentric

Fig.1

2. MUAP parameters[1]

The motor unit action potential (MUAP) from a voluntarily contracting muscle contains the summed electrical activity of all the single muscle fibers belonging to a particular motor unit.

Normal parameters for *amplitude* and *duration* will depend on the needle used, muscle studied, and age of the pt. Using a concentric needle, a rough range of normal amplitudes for limb muscles might be 160-460µV; for durations, the range might be about 6-15ms. MUAPs for the elderly are slightly larger than those of young adults.

Aging and reduced temperatures can increase phasicity. A MUAP with ≥5 phases is *polyphasic*.

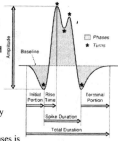

Fig.2

3. Insertional activity[1]

Brief (<300ms), crisp bursts of electrical potentials following quick movements of a needle electrode through muscle are consistent with "normal insertional activity."

Minimal or no electrical activity following the same movements is consistent with the qualitative term "decreased insertional activity." The duration of spikes is <300ms. The cause may be fibrotic muscle tissue or periodic paralysis.

"Increased insertional activity" is characterized by prolonged (i.e., >300-500ms) electrical activity after the cessation of needle movement. The pathologic significance of this phenomenon, however, is unclear. It may represent denervation or myopathy, or it may be a normal variant.

References: 1. **Dumitru D**, ed.: *Electrodiagnostic Medicine*, 2nd ed. Hanley & Belfus, 2002. **Fig.1** courtesy of **Oh SJ**: *Principles of Clinical EMG: Case Studies*. LWW, 1998. **Fig.2** courtesy of **Dumitru D**, ed.: *EDx Medicine*, 2nd ed. Hanley & Belfus, 2002.

80

4. Spontaneous activity[1]

Endplate activity

a. Monopolar needle electrode located in relaxed muscle.

b. MEPPs - Miniature endplate potentials are negative monophasic waves firing irregularly at 150Hz with 0.5-2ms duration and 10-50μV amplitude. MEPPs represent the spontaneous release of single quanta of ACh (prejunctional activity) with a local subthreshold postsynaptic response. They sound like a "seashell held to the ear."

c. Endplate spikes are initially negative biphasic waves firing irregularly at 1-100Hz with 3-4ms duration and <1mV amplitude. They represent the depolarization of a single muscle fiber 2° to a suprathreshold endplate potential generated by the needle electrode. They can have initial positive spikes if the needle is out of endplate zone. They sound like "bacon sputtering."

d. MMEPs and endplate spikes.

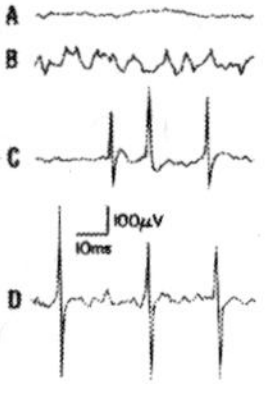

Fig.1

Fibrillations, positive sharp waves (PSWs)

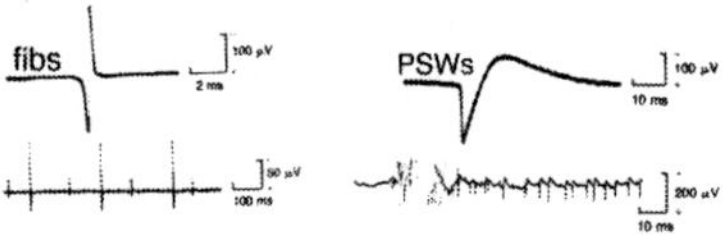

Fibs and PSWs are the electric activity associated with spontaneously contracting muscle.

fibs

PSWs

They are associated with an alteration in the resting membrane potential of denervated muscle to a less negative value, approaching w/in several mV of threshold.

Fibs are regularly firing initially positive biphasic waves of short duration (<5 ms) and small amplitude (<1 mV) that sound like "rain on a tin roof." They represent spontaneously firing single muscle fibers. PSWs have negative phases with a lower amplitude and longer duration (10-100 ms). PSWs sound like "dull pops." The clinical significance of fibs and PSWs is the same.

Fibs and PSWs are graded as:
1+   transient following needle movement at 2 sites
2+   occasional at rest in >2 sites
3+   present at rest in most sites
4+   abundant, almost filling the screen at all sites

Fig.2

Fasciculation potentials

Fascics are the electrically summated voltage of random, non-voluntary depolarizing muscle fibers belonging to a single motor unit. They are associated with motor neuron disease, chronic radiculopathy, peripheral neuropathy, and thyrotoxicosis. They may be seen in normal individuals under certain conditions, e.g., stress, fatigue, caffeine-intake.

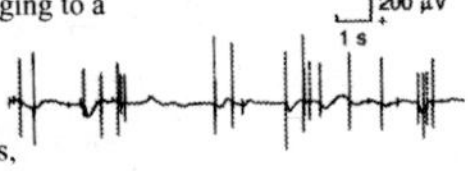

Fig.3

Complex repetitive discharges (CRDs)

CRDs are caused by ephaptic transmission from one muscle fiber to an adjacent fiber. They may occur spontaneously or follow needle movements. They are characterized by runs of spike patterns that repeat at 0.3 to 150 Hz. They sound like a "motorcycle" or "heavy machinery."

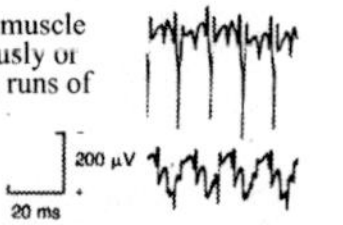

Fig.4

References: 1. **Dumitru D**, ed.: *Electrodiagnostic Medicine*, 2nd ed. Hanley & Belfus, 2002. **Fig.1** courtesy of **Dumitru D**, ed.: *Electrodiagnostic Medicine*, 2nd ed. Hanley & Belfus, 2002. **Figs.2,3,4** courtesy of **DeLisa JA**, ed.: *Manual of Nerve Conduction Velocity and Clinical Neurophysiology*, 3rd ed. Raven Press, 1994.

Myotonic discharges

Myotonic discharges are associated with membrane instability and are seen in many clinical conditions, e.g., myopathy, myotonia. They have a waxing and waning amplitude and frequency and sound like a "dive bomber."

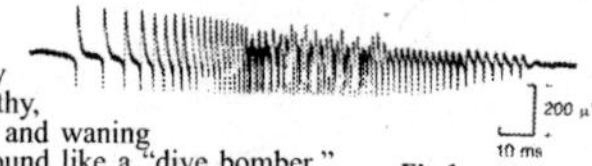

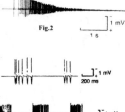

Fig.1

Neuromyotonia

Neuromyotonia is a syndrome of continuous muscle fiber activity manifested as muscle rippling and stiffness, e.g., Isaac's syndrome.

Fig.2

Myokymic potentials

Myokymic potentials are due to the ephaptic firing of MUAPs from the anterior horn cell or any portion of the peripheral nerve. There are irregular bursts of abnormal motor units at 0.1-10Hz, with interburst silence, unaffected by voluntary activity. They sound like the "sputtering of a low-powered motor boat engine" or "marching soldiers." They are seen with radiation plexopathy, MS, brainstem neoplasms, syringomyelia, radiculopathy, uremia, and thyrotoxicosis.

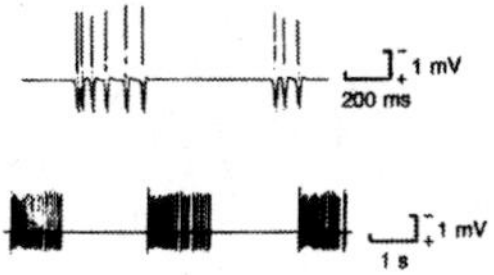

Fig.3

5. Motor Unit Analysis

The *recruitment ratio* is the rate of the fastest-firing MUAP divided by the # of different MUAPs on screen. In normal individuals, this ratio should be 5-10. Thus, as the 1st MUAP increases its firing rate and reaches ~10Hz, the 2nd MUAP will be recruited and begin to fire.

If the recruitment ratio is <5, too many motor units are being recruited for the generated force. This is increased or "early" recruitment, which is consistent with a *myopathic process*. Other motor units are being recruited to compensate for the small, weak initially-recruited motor units.

If the ratio is >10, not enough MUAPs are being recruited for the generated force. This is decreased or "late" recruitment, which is consistent with a LMN disease or *neurogenic process*. Motor units have been lost due to denervation.

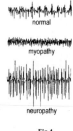

The *interference pattern* is the electrical activity recorded with voluntary contractions. An interference pattern with a moderate voluntary contraction is pictured at right. When a full interference pattern is noted with minimal contraction, this is described as a *myopathic pattern*.

Patterns associated with LMN disease, or *neurogenic patterns*, have a "picket fence" appearance with gaps on maximal contraction.

Fig.4

Figs.1,2 courtesy of **Goodgold J**: *Electrodiagnosis of Neuromuscular Diseases*, 2nd ed. Williams & Wilkins, 1977. **Fig.3** courtesy of **DeLisa JA**, ed.: *Manual of Nerve Conduction Velocity and Clinical Neurophysiology*, 3rd ed. Raven Press, 1994. **Fig.4** courtesy of **Johnson E**, ed.: *Practical Electromyography*, 3rd ed. Williams & Wilkins, 1997.

C. Basic EDx Principles and Guidelines*

*Many protocols exist. Refer to the American Academy of Electrodiagnostic Medicine (AAEM) guidelines for detailed protocols. The following includes generalized approaches and/or *examples* of some protocols, most of which have been simplified for brevity.

1. Limitations of EDx[1]

Some limitations of EDx include 1) NCS selectively studies only large myelinated fibers and does not define diseases in smaller nerves. 2) Motor conduction studies are not available for most proximal or most distal segments of nerves. 3) Sensory NCS only evaluate post-ganglionic, not preganglionic lesions. Sensory NCS do not correlate with pain and are not useful for evaluating conduction block due to temporal dispersion and excessive cancellation. 4) Needle EMG evaluates mainly small motor units and not the larger units recruited later. Needle EMG provides pathophysiologic information only, not etiology.

2. Myopathy

a. Perform one motor and one sensory NCS to determine if there is concurrent peripheral nerve involvement. Myopathy alone should not produce abnormalities in NCS, although CMAPs may be reduced.

b. Perform EMGs in two limbs, proximally and distally. Look for early MUAP recruitment, ↑ polyphasia, and small-amplitude short-duration MUAPs. The thoracic paraspinals may provide increased sensitivity.

c. May also perform repetitive nerve stimulation to r/o a NMJ disorder.

3. Neuromuscular junction (NMJ) disorders

a. Perform a sensory NCS in a clinically involved limb; results should be normal. Examine ulnar motor nerve conduction to the ADM, with F wave analysis. Baseline CMAP amplitudes may be normal or ↓ in postsynaptic disorders (e.g., MG) or very low in presynaptic disorders (e.g., LEMS).

b. Perform repetitive nerve stimulation (RNS) studies. Findings consistent with a NMJ disorder include post-tetanic facilitation, post-tetanic exhaustion, and decrement on slow RNS (2-3Hz). A dx of MG is supported by a mild increment on fast RNS (>24Hz) or after exercise. A dx of LEMS is supported by a large increment on fast RNS or after exercise. If the initial muscle studied is unrevealing, RNS of a more proximal nerve (e.g., spinal accessory, facial n.) should be considered.

c. If a decrement >10% is not noted on RNS, single fiber EMG of the EDC or a more proximal muscle can be considered. Findings consistent with, but not specific for, NMJ disorders include increased jitter (see right) and blocking.

normal

d. Perform EMG of at least one distal and one proximal muscle, primarily to r/o other disorders. Denervation potentials are rare except in long-term severe disease. Rapidly firing, small-amplitude, short-duration MUAPs are not specific for NMJ disorders, but may be seen.

Increased jitter

Reference: 1. **Oh-Park M**: General principles of electrodiagnosis. In **O'Young BJ**, ed.: *PMR Secrets*, 2nd ed. Hanley & Belfus, 2002. Figure courtesy of **Rowland LP**, ed.: *Merritt's Neurology*, 10th ed. LWW, 2000.

4. Nerve injury classification, electrophysiology[1]

Seddon	Sunderland	Pathology/Prognosis
Neurapraxia	Type I	Local myelin injury and conduction block. Axon intact. No Wallerian degeneration. Recovery in weeks to months.
Axonotmesis	Type II	Wallerian degeneration and disruption of axonal continuity. Endoneurial tubes, perineurium, epineurium intact. Good prognosis since the intact endoneurium allows regenerating axons to grow back w/o misdirection, provided the distance between lesion and end organ is not too long.
	Type III	Axons and endoneurium discontinuous. Perineurium and epineurium intact. Poor prognosis. Surgery may be required.
	Type IV	Loss of axonal continuity, endoneurium, and perineurium. Epineurium intact. Poor prognosis. Surgery necessary.
Neurotmesis	Type V	Severance of entire nerve. Prognosis guarded and dependent upon nature of injury and local factors. Surgical modification of nerve ends required.

Conduction block (CB) - CB is the failure of action potentials to propagate across a lesion, whereas conduction is possible below the lesion (i.e., NCS below the lesion are normal). Large myelinated and motor fibers are usually more affected than unmyelinated or sensory fibers.

When recording across the lesion, CMAP amplitudes are diminished. Criteria vary, but Dumitru suggests a 30% drop for the UEx and 40% for the LEx, provided that the drops are not due to excessive temporal dispersion. Others have suggested a 20% criterion for any limb. Conduction velocity is *not* a reliable indicator in the assessment of CB.

Demyelination (DM) - DM may manifest as decreased NCV, conduction block, or both. If the CMAP amplitude is >80% of the lower limit of normal (LLN), a NCV of <80% of the LLN suggests DM. If the CMAP amplitude is <80% of the LLN, a NCV of <70% of the LLN suggests DM.

Axonal loss - A loss of CMAP amplitude (when recording distally to the presumed lesion site) that persists >6-7days after injury suggests axonal loss. Side-to-side comparisons may be more reliable than using normal values. Side-to-side differences of 10-20% may be w/in normal variation.

It may *not* be possible to distinguish axonal loss from CB w/in 7 days of injury since distal CMAPs may be obtainable in both scenarios.

Reference: **1. Dumitru D.** ed.: *Electrodiagnostic Medicine*, 2nd ed. Hanley & Belfus, 2002.

5. Selected mononeuropathies

Bell's palsy - Compare side-to-side facial NCS. CMAP amplitude during the first two wks is the most reliable indicator of prognosis (particularly after days 5-7). A >90% loss of CMAP amplitude suggests a prolonged and incomplete recovery. The more quickly the 90% loss is achieved, the worse the outcome. The blink reflex is *not* useful for prognosis.

Ulnar neuropathy at the elbow (UNE) - Obtain ulnar ADM CMAPs, stimulating at the wrist, and below/above the elbow. The elbow should be in 90° flexion; the across-elbow distance should be

10cm. Evidence for UNE includes an across-elbow NCV >10m/s slower than the NCV in the forearm; an across-elbow drop in CMAP amplitude of >20%; and an above-elbow CMAP waveform different than below the elbow.

If inconclusive, NCSs with the FDI as motor point or an inching study at the elbow can be considered.

Median neuropathy at the wrist/carpal tunnel syndrome (CTS)[1,2]

a. Obtain a sensory NCS of the median n. across the wrist, and if the latency is abnormal, compare with another sensory study in the same limb. A 14cm median latency that is more than 0.5m greater than the ulnar latency suggests CTS. If both are abnormal, a proximal lesion may be responsible. If the initial median NCS across the wrist has a conduction distance >8cm and the results are normal, perform a median NCS over a short (7-8cm) distance or compare median to ipsilateral radial or ulnar conductions. If equivocal, median inching studies can also be considered.

b. Median motor NCS should be compared to another ipsilateral motor NCS. A needle EMG study is optional. EMG has low sensitivity in early CTS, but may detect aggressive lesions or a concomitant cervical radiculopathy.

6. Selected anomalous innervations[2]

Martin-Gruber anastomosis (MGA) - The MGA is a common forearm anastomosis between the median and ulnar nerves. Incidence is 7.7-34%; 68% of cases have b/l MGAs. In 91% of cases, there is a communicating branch from the anterior interosseus n. to the ulnar n. Clinically, if there is an ulnar lesion *proximal* to this communication, ulnar-supplied hand intrinsics may still be functional because of the MGA fibers.

With a MGA, the median n. APB CMAP will be larger when stimulated proximally than distally. This is because proximal, but not distal, stimulation activates the MGA-innervated muscles (e.g., deep head of FPB and adductor pollicis). Volume conduction from these muscles increases the apparent CMAP amplitude and causes an initially positive deflection.

If a MGA and median neuropathy at the wrist are present concomitantly, distal median n. latencies will be prolonged while proximal latencies may be normal (due to volume conduction of MGA/ulnar-innervated muscles). NCVs calculated from these latencies may be artificially very high.

Accessory deep peroneal nerve (ADPN) - The ADPN arises from the superficial peroneal n., travels posterior to the lateral malleolus, and innervates the EDB. Incidence may be as high as 28%; 57% have b/l involvement.

An EDB CMAP that is larger with proximal (fibular head) stimulation than distal stimulation suggests an ADPN. An EDB response with posterior lateral malleolus stimulation is confirmatory. Caution, however, should be taken to r/o volume conduction from tibial-innervated foot intrinsics (the latter may have an initial positive deflection).

Failure to recognize an ADPN may lead a clinician to believe that a complete lesion of the deep peroneal n. (e.g., no tibialis anterior or EHL) is incomplete due to voluntary EDB activation.

Reference: **1. Limke JC**: CTS and/or median neuropathy at the wrist. In O'Young BJ, ed.: *PMR Secrets*, 2nd ed. Hanley & Belfus, 2002. **2. Dumitru D**, ed.: *Electrodiagnostic Medicine*, 2nd ed. Hanley & Belfus, 2002.

7. Polyneuropathy[1,2]

a. Perform sural, superficial peroneal, median and ulnar sensory NCS and peroneal, tibial, median, and ulnar motor NCS on at least one side. F waves should be performed on all motor nerves studied if a demyelinating process is suspected. Definite abnormalities should be followed by evaluation of the opposite extremity. With prominent cranial nerve involvement, facial motor NCS and/or blink reflex studies should be considered.

b. Perform EMG of paraspinals, 1 UEx, and 1 LEx. EMG substantiates the impression of axonal loss (e.g., ↑ insertional activity, fibs, PSWs, ↓ recruitment, and possibly ↑ MUAP amplitude/duration) or demyelination (e.g., ↓ recruitment w/o membrane instability or MUAP changes).

Classification and EDx findings in polyneuropathies:

Uniform demyelinating, mixed sensorimotor polyneuropathy (e.g., Charcot Marie Tooth [CMT]/HMSN I, III, IV). NCS: reduced NCV (<80-90% of lower limit of normal), no conduction block, prolonged F, minimal/no temporal dispersion. EMG: denervation potentials and ↓ recruitment.

Segmental demyelinating motor > sensory polyneuropathy (e.g., AIDP, CIDP, multifocal neuropathy with motor conduction block). NCS: NCV slowing, temporal dispersion, prolonged/absent F, patchy sensory studies. EMG: abnormal spontaneous activity, ↑ polyphasia and MUAP amplitude. *Note:* The North American GBS Study Group reports that the earliest EMG change in AIDP is F wave prolongation, while others report that it is conduction block. In AIDP, a markedly ↓ CMAP amplitude (<10-20% of the lower limit of normal) from an intrinsic hand muscle recorded at about 3-4wks correlates with poor outcome.

Axonal loss, motor > sensory polyneuropathy (e.g., CMT/HMSN II, acute intermittent porphyria, acute axonal GBS, lead neuropathy, hypoglycemia). NCS: ↓ motor and sensory amplitudes, with intact NCVs until late in the disease process. EMG: evidence of denervation.

Axonal loss sensory neuropathy (e.g., carcinomatous sensory neuropathy, HSAN, Fisher variant of GBS, Sjögren's syndrome, Fredreich's ataxia). NCS: ↓ or absent SNAPs with normal motor NCS. EMG: typically normal.

Axonal loss, mixed sensorimotor polyneuropathy (e.g., multiple myeloma, amyloidosis, vasculitic neuropathies, critical illness neuropathy, gouty neuropathy, most toxic [e.g., EtOH] and metabolic polyneuropathies). NCS: initially ↓ sensory amplitudes, with NCV generally normal until there is a substantial ↓ in amplitudes. EMG: can show distal denervation.

Mixed axonal loss and demyelinating sensorimotor polyneuropathy (e.g., diabetic neuropathy, uremia). NCS: ↓ sensory amplitudes with moderate NCV slowing. Motor studies show similar findings later.

Asymmetric motor and sensory polyneuropathy (e.g., mononeuropathy multiplex). This is characterized by asymmetric/ multifocal clinical/EDx findings. Mononeuropathy multiplex is classically due to polyarteritis nodosa.

References: **1. Donofrio PD**: AAEM Minimonograph #34: Polyneuropathy: Classification by NCS and EMG. *Muscle Nerve* 1990;13:889-903. **2. Dumitru D**: *Electrodiagnostic Medicine,* 2nd ed. Hanley & Belfus, 2002.

8. Selected Plexopathies

Plexus lesions distal to the DRG can lead to Wallerian degeneration with complete SNAP loss w/in 7-10days. In nerve root avulsions, sensory NCS may remain normal because the lesion is proximal to the DRG. CMAP amplitude loss is indicative of conduction block or axonal loss. Late responses are of limited utility in a plexopathy study. EMG abnormalities are vital in the localization of the lesion and determination of the injury's extent. SSEPs can be useful in assessing brachial neuropathies.

Neoplastic vs. radiation-induced (XRT) plexopathy - Neoplastic plexopathies are typically caused by metastatic tumors (e.g., Pancoast tumors from lung, breast metastases via lymphatic spread) and typically affect the lower plexus. Symptoms include aching shoulder/scapular pain, weakness/wasting of the hand intrinsic muscles, medial upper limb paresthesias, and Horner's Syndrome. CMAP loss may be more severe than in XRT plexopathy. Myokymic discharges are very rare.

XRT plexopathy is due to fibrosis in the vasa nervosum and ischemic axonal and Schwann cell damage. Symptoms may arise months to years post exposure and are directly related to XRT dose. Classically, XRT plexopathy is said to be *less painful* than neoplastic plexopathy. Key EDx findings c/w XRT plexopathy are *myokymic discharges* and, to a lesser extent, fasciculations. The earliest finding may be a ↓ median SNAP amplitude. Despite these findings, differentiating XRT from neoplastic plexopathies may be extremely difficult or impossible. Imaging is recommended.

Thoracic outlet syndrome (TOS) - "True neurogenic" TOS typically affects the lower plexus. The majority of cases have a cervical rib. Classic NCS findings include a normal latency, low amplitude medial antebrachial cutaneous SNAP and median CMAP. These are more affected than the ulnar SNAP and CMAP, which can be variable. The median SNAP is normal. EMG can show PSWs/fibs, reduced/late recruitment, and large amplitude, long duration MUAPs in the APB. Paraspinals are spared, indicating that the lesion is distal to the origin of the posterior primary rami.

9. Radiculopathy

SNAP amplitudes and latencies should be normal in radiculopathy. CMAP amplitudes may be ↓, although this is *not* usually the case. A prolonged onset latency of the H reflex may be useful in diagnosing C6/C7 or S1 radiculopathies, provided there is an absence of findings along the nerve(s) distal to the root and normal responses are found in the asymptomatic limbs. F waves are of minimal utility in the study of radiculopathies.

Needle EMG should be performed in a sufficient number of muscles such that a radiculopathy can be defined or would be most likely (3 muscles of the same myotome with different peripheral innervation). MUAPs may have ↑ duration, amplitude, and polyphasicity with ↓ recruitment. PSW/fibs are generally said to appear in the paraspinals first (~5-7days post-injury), then peripherally in 3-6wks[1]. With reinnervation, they may disappear after 3mos. The appearance/disappearance of membrane instability on EMG may not correlate with this time-frame, however, because pts' reporting of the onset of symptoms is not highly reliable[2].

The sensitivity of EMG for detecting radiculopathy is about 50-80% for lumbosacral lesions and 60-70% for cervical[1]. A radiculopathy cannot be ruled out before 2-4wks post-injury, although an EDx study during this window may be helpful in ruling out pre-existing pathology.

Cervical radiculopathies are likely to be due to bony factors or ligamentous hypertrophy. The most commonly affected root is C7 (incidence, 31-81%), followed by C6 (19-25%)[1]. C8 and C5 are less commonly affected. Thoracic radiculopathies can be due to diabetes mellitus, but are very rare.

Lumbosacral radiculopathies are likely due to disc herniation. The majority of lesions involve the L5 and S1 roots. L4 radiculopathies are less common, while L1-3 involvement is rare. A L5 radiculopathy is the most common unilateral/unilevel radiculopathy.

Sample radiculopathy screens[4,5]:

CERVICAL	Root	Nerve	LUMBAR	Root	Nerve
Deltoid	**C5-C6**	Axillary	Vast Med	**L2-L3-L4**	Femoral
Triceps	**C6-C7-C8**	Radial	Tib Ant	**L4-L5**-S1	Deep Per
Pron Teres	**C6-C7**	Median	Tib Post	(L4)-**L5**-S1	Tibial
EDC	**C7-C8**	Radial	Bcp Fem, SH	**L5-S1**-S2	Com Per
APB	**C8**-T1	Median	Med Gastroc	**L5-S1-S2**	Tibial
Paraspinals		Post rami	Paraspinals		Post rami

This screen had an identification rate (*not* sensitivity) of up to 99% w/ neuropathic findings[4].

This screen had an identification rate (*not* sensitivity) of up to 100% w/ neuropathic findings[5].

References: **1. Dimitru D**, ed.: *EDx Medicine*, 2nd ed. Hanley & Belfus, 2002. **2. Dillingham TR**: Cervical paraspinal muscle abnormalities and symptom duration: a multivariate analysis. *Muscle Nerve* 1998;21:640-2. **3. Dillingham TR**: Radiculopathies. In O'Young BJ, ed.: *PMR Secrets*, 2nd ed. Hanley & Belfus, 2002. **4. Dillingham TR**: Identification of cervical radiculopathies: Optimizing the EMG screen. *Am J PMR* 2001;80:84-91. **5. Dillingham TR**: Identifying lumbosacral radiculopathies: an optimal EMG screen. *Am J PMR* 2000;79:496-503.

10. Selected Neuronopathies

Amyotrophic lateral sclerosis (ALS) - Clinical signs and symptoms are consistent with a combined UMN and LMN lesion.

Lambert criteria[1]: 1) normal sensory NCVs; 2) normal motor NCVs, except when the amplitude is abnormal (in which case NCVs should remain >70% of the mean expected NCV); 3) Fibs/PSWs and fasciculations in ≥3 limbs, with the bulbar muscles counting as a "limb"; 4) EMG shows late recruitment with ↑ MUAP duration and amplitude.

Post Polio Syndrome (PPS) - About 25-50% of pts who suffer paralysis or paresis due to polio will go on to develop additional dysfunction roughly 30yrs later and are said to have PPS. The **Halstead and Rossi** criteria include the onset of two or more of the following: worsened fatigue, muscle and joint pain, new weakness/atrophy, and functional loss or cold intolerance w/o another explanatory medical dx in the setting of confirmed paralytic polio with ≥15 years of neurologic and functional stability[2].

There are no pathognomonic EDx findings, but NCS may show normal SNAPs and motor NCVs if CMAPs have not been obliterated by atrophy. EMG may reveal ↑ amplitude, ↑ duration MUAPs with ↓ recruitment.

References: **1. Lambert EH**: EMG in ALS. In Norris FH, ed.: *Motor Neuron Diseases*. Grunc& Stratton, 1969. **2. Halstead LS**. ed.: *Research and clinical aspects of the late effects of poliomyelitis*. March of Dimes Birth Defects Foundation, 1987.

XVI. Traumatic Brain Injury (TBI)

A. Introduction and Epidemiology

Accurate *incidence* is difficult to assess since many who suffer mild TBI are not seen by physicians. Estimates for all severities of TBI range from 500,000 to 2 million episodes/yr in the U.S.[1,2] The majority are classified as mild injuries. About 52,000 cases annually are fatal[2]. There is a bimodal age distribution with the highest peak at 15-24yrs (200-225/100,000) and a second peak at 65-75yrs (200/100,000)[1]. The ♂:♀ ratio is at least 2:1, although this ratio decreases with increasing age[1,3].

About 44,000 people/yr survive TBI with moderate to severe physical or neurobehavioral sequelae[1]. The NIH estimates that between 2.5-6.5 million Americans are living with TBI-related disabilities[2]. The socio-economic impact is enormous. Total lifetime costs for all persons who incurred a TBI in 1985 in the U.S. have been estimated to be $37.8billion[1].

Motor vehicle accidents (MVAs) account for about half of all TBIs[2]. Falls are the second most common cause of TBI in the very young and elderly[2]. Violence-related incidents account for ~20% of TBI, with roughly half of these related to firearms[2]. Sports/recreational activities account for 3% of hospitalized cases; however many cases are mild and may go unreported[2]. Fifty-one percent of TBI cases in the NIDRR TBI Model Systems database were legally intoxicated (EtOH) at time of injury[3].

References: **1. Whyte J**: Rehabilitation of the patient with TBI. In **DeLisa J**, ed.: *Rehabilitation Medicine: Principles and Practice.* 3rd ed. Lippincott-Raven, 1998. **2. Ragnarsson KT**: NIH Consensus Development Panel on Rehabilitation of Persons with TBI. *JAMA* 1999;282:974-83. **3. Gordon WA**: Demographic and social characteristics of the TBI Model System Database. *J Head Trauma Rehabil* 1993;8:26-33.

B. Pathophysiology of Primary Injury

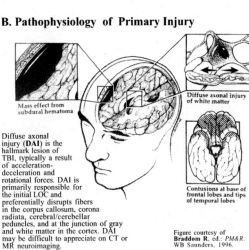

Mass effect from subdural hematoma

Diffuse axonal injury of white matter

Diffuse axonal injury **(DAI)** is the hallmark lesion of TBI, typically a result of acceleration-deceleration and rotational forces. DAI is primarily responsible for the initial LOC and preferentially disrupts fibers in the corpus callosum, corona radiata, cerebral/cerebellar peduncles, and at the junction of gray and white matter in the cortex. DAI may be difficult to appreciate on CT or MR neuroimaging.

Contusions at base of frontal lobes and tips of temporal lobes

Figure courtesy of **Braddom R**, ed.: *PM&R.* WB Saunders, 1996.

C. TBI-Related Concomitant Injuries

Most pts admitted to hospitals with TBI have concomitant injuries; *fractures* and *cranial nerve injuries* are most common. C-spine, pelvis, hips, and knee films are appropriate screening studies. A bone scan at 7-10days post-injury to detect occult fxs is not unreasonable. CNs VII and III are most commonly injured. CN I is also commonly injured; its incidence, however, is unknown since it is not commonly tested. Complaints of headache and dizziness are often seen.

D. Acute Treatment of TBI

Moderate *hypothermia* (33°C x24hr) instituted acutely may reduce neuronal damage due to excitotoxicity and improve long-term function in some subgroups of severe TBI pts[1], although true efficacy is not clear. The use of *neuroprotective agents* (e.g., glutamate receptor antagonists, free radical scavengers, Ca-channel blockers) in TBI is under investigation. Some agents hold promise; a phase III trial of the antioxidant *pegorgotein*, however, failed to demonstrate improved outcomes versus placebo[2].

Increased intracranial pressures (ICPs) with reduced cerebral perfusion may first be managed with elevation of the head of the bed. *Hyperventilation* is a secondary measure. *Barbiturates* are thought to reduce cerebral metabolic rate and lipid peroxidation; their role in reducing elevated ICPs is controversial. *Mannitol* is used for increased ICPs due to edema.

References: 1. **Marion DW**: Treatment of traumatic brain injury with moderate hypothermia. *NEJM* 1997;336:540-546. 2. **Young B**: Effects of pegorgotein on neurologic outcome of patients with severe head injury-a multicenter, randomized controlled trial. *JAMA* 1996;276:538-43.

E. Attributes of Coma, Vegetative State, and the Minimally Conscious State[1,2]

Clinical feature	Coma	Vegetative state	Minimally conscious state
spontaneous eye opening	no	yes	yes
sleep-wake cycle	no	resumes	abnormal to WNL
arousal	no	sluggish, poorly sustained	obtunded to WNL
evidence of perception, communication ability, or purposeful motor activity	no	no	reproducible, but inconsistent
visual tracking	no	none, but may have roving eye movements	often intact
yes/no responses, gestures, verbalizations	no	no	none to unreliable, inconsistent

References: 1. **Giacino JT**: Development of practice guidelines for assessment and management of the vegetative and minimally conscious states. *J Head Trauma Rehabil* 1997;12:79-89. 2. **Giacino JT**: The vegetative and minimally conscious states: a comparison of clinical features and functional outcome. *J Head Trauma Rehabil* 1997;12:36-51.

F. Glasgow Coma Scale

Eye opening (E)		Best motor (M)		Best verbal (V)	
spontaneous	4	obeys verbal commands	6	oriented, able to converse	5
to speech	3	localizes painful stimulus	5	disoriented, confused	4
to pain	2	flexion withdrawal	4	inappropriate words	3
no eye opening	1	abnormal flexion response	3	incomprehensible sounds	2
		extensor response	2	no verbal response	1
		no motor response	1		

Reference: **Teasdale G**: Assessment of coma and impaired consciousness. *Lancet* 1974;2:81-4.

G. TBI Severity and Prognosis

	Level of Severity		
Index	Mild (concussion)	Moderate	Severe
GCS	13-15	9-12	≤8
LOC	<30 min	≤ 24 hrs	>24 hrs
duration of PTA	0-24 hrs	1-7 days	>7 days
permanent neurologic and neuro-ψ sequelae	none likely	some likely; pts often quite functional	severe deficits likely

The GCS is a strong predictor of functional outcome. Duration of LOC is also predictive. If the pt is unconscious at 1mo post-TBI, there is ~50% likelihood of regaining consciousness by 1yr post-injury[1]. Prognosis for non-traumatic brain injury (e.g., anoxia) is usually worse.

Post traumatic amnesia (PTA), a strong predictor of outcome in moderate to severe TBI, is defined as the period after TBI in which new information is not incorporated into long-term memory. PTA can be assessed with the *Galveston Orientation and Amnesia Test* (GOAT), which is scored from 0-100 (≥75 is considered normal). The end of PTA is marked by a GOAT score of ≥75 on at least 2 consecutive days. An alternative to the GOAT is the *Westmead* PTA scale.

Reference: **1.** Sazbon L: Outcome in 134 pts with prolonged posttraumatic unawareness. Parameters determining late recovery of consciousness. *J Neurosurg* 1990;72:75-80.

H. Rancho Los Amigos Cognitive Functioning Scale

I.	No response to any stimuli
II.	Generalized response to stimulation
III.	Localized response to stimuli
IV.	Confused and agitated
V.	Confused with inappropriate behavior (non-agitated)
VI.	Confused but appropriate behavior
VII.	Automatic and appropriate behavior
VIII.	Purposeful and appropriate behavior

The Rancho Los Amigos (RLA) scale is a descriptive scale primarily used to facilitate communication among members of the rehabilitation team. An orderly progression from level I-VIII during recovery from TBI has *not* been demonstrated scientifically.
Reference: *Rehabilitation of the head-injured adult: comprehensive physical management.* Professional Staff Association, Rancho Los Amigos Hospital, 1979.

I. Issues in TBI Rehabilitation

Agitation - Medical etiologies (e.g., infection, metabolic abnormalities, hypoxemia, seizures, hydrocephalus, hematoma, cerebral edema) should be suspected and ruled out first. *Pain* may present as agitation, or it may worsen agitation. *Tx* includes behavioral and environmental modifications (i.e., Vail bed). *Carbamezepine, trazodone,* and *amantidine* were preferred over haloperidol, benzodiazepines, and propranolol in a survey of TBI experts[1].

Dysautonomia - A clinical syndrome of increased HR, BP, RR, fever, dystonia, and sweating. *Tx* options include β-blockers, NSAIDs, and morphine. Bromocriptine may be used for central fevers.

Endocrine - *SIADH* is common in the acute period and is characterized by euvolemia, hyponatremia, low BUN (<10 mg/dL), and ↓blood and ↑urine (>150 mOsm/kg) osmolality. *Tx* is water restriction (e.g., 1L/day) or a high salt diet with furosemide. (Beware of central pontine myelinolysis due to overrapid correction of hyponatremia.) *Salt wasting* may be more common and should be corrected (e.g., NaCl tabs, IV NS). *Diabetes insipidus* is rare.

Pediatric TBI - Prognosis for recovery of consciousness and mobility after severe TBI may be better than for adults. Overall functional outcome may be poorer, however, due to the adverse effects on learning.

Pharmacotherapy of arousal - General arousal and alertness may improve with increased dopaminergic activity (e.g., *bromocriptine, amantadine*) and somewhat less consistently with increased serotoninergic activity (e.g., *trazodone, sertraline*). *Methylphenidate* is thought to improve arousal by facilitating norepinephrine and dopamine release in the brainstem. Similar helpful stimulants include *Adderall* (mixed amphetamine salts) and *modafinil*. Some medications may impede recovery in the TBI pt and should be avoided if possible, e.g., benzodiazepines, haloperidol, phenytoin.

Post-traumatic epilepsy (PTE) - PTE is noted in 5-7% of all hospitalized TBI pts, 11% of severe non-penetrating TBI, and 35-50% of penetrating TBI[2]. Early seizures (during the 1st wk post-TBI) increase the risk of late seizures (after 1st wk). Prophylactic *phenytoin* reduces early seizures after severe TBI (3.6% vs. 14.2% for placebo), but benefit is not noted between day 8 and 2 yrs post-TBI[3]. For penetrating TBI, the efficacy of PTE prophylaxis beyond day 8 is not clearly established[4]. *Carbamezepine* and *valproic acid* are the preferred agents for *tx* of PTE. Tx duration for late seizures is not clearly established; many clinicians stop after 1-2 seizure-free years.

Post-traumatic headache (PTHA) - PTHA is commonly seen and it may present as a tension-type or vascular-type of HA. Myofascial neck pain and other causes of HA should be suspected and treated if present. Persistent PTHA may necessitate further work up to rule out intracranial pathology.

Post-traumatic hyperthermia (PTHT) - First, medical etiologies should be ruled out (e.g., infection, spasticity, heterotopic ossification, drug fevers). PTHT of cerebral origin is rare. *Tx* includes cooling blankets, dantrolene, and antipyretics.

References: **1. Fugate LP:** A survey of the Brain Injury Interest Group of the AAPMR. *Arch PMR* 1997;78:924-8. **2. Yablon SA:** Posttraumatic seizures. *Arch PMR* 1993;74:983-1001. **3. Temkin NR:** A randomized double-blind study of phenytoin for the prevention of posttraumatic seizures. *NEJM* 1990;323:497-502. **4. Brain Injury SIG of the AAPM&R:** Practice parameter: antiepileptic drug tx of posttraumatic seizures. *Arch PMR* 1998;79:594-7.

XVII. STROKE

A. Introduction, Epidemiology, and Risk Factors

A stroke is defined by the WHO as the rapid development of clinical signs of cerebral dysfunction, with signs lasting at least 24hrs or leading to death with no apparent cause other than that of vascular origin[1]. There are ~700,000 new strokes/year in the U.S., with ~150,000 deaths/year w/in 1mo after the stroke[2]. There are approximately 4 million stroke survivors, and many have residual functional deficits[2]. Stroke is the 2nd leading cause of disability after arthritis and the most common cause of severe disability[2].

The two major types of stroke are *ischemic* (~83%) and *hemorrhagic* (17%)[3]. Further categorized, 32% are embolic, 31% large vessel thrombotic, 20% small vessel thrombotic, 10% intracerebral hemorrhagic, and 7% subarachnoid hemorrhagic[3]. The Framingham Heart Study data revealed 30 day survival to be 73-81% following cerebral infarction and 36% after intracerebral hemorrhage[4], although survival figures vary widely in the literature and have generally been improving with time.

Males, African-Americans, and the elderly are at increased risk of developing stroke. Modifiable risk factors include HTN, DM, hypercholesterolemia, hyperhomocysteinemia, hypercoaguable states, heart disease, carotid arteriosclerosis, substance abuse, obesity, and a sedentary lifestyle.

B. Selected Ischemic Stroke Syndromes

MCA - Deficits can include c/l hemiplegia/hypesthesia (face and arm worse than leg), c/l homonymous hemianopia, and i/l gaze preference.

With *dominant* hemisphere involvement, receptive aphasia (inferior div. of MCA to Wernicke's area) and/or expressive aphasia (sup. div. of MCA to Broca's area) can occur, but classically, pts can learn from demonstration and mistakes. *Gerstmann's syndrome* (parietal lobe) consists of asomatognosia (right-left confusion), dyscalculia, finger agnosia, and dysgraphia.

With *non-dominant* hemisphere involvement, spatial dyspraxia and c/l hemineglect may be seen; insight/judgment are often affected (likely to need supervision); ADL recovery is often said to be slower.

ACA - Deficits can include c/l hemiplegia/hypesthesia (leg worse than arm; face and hand spared), alien hand/hand syndrome, urinary incontinence, gait apraxia, abulia (inability to make decisions), perseveration, amnesia, paratonic rigidity (*Gegenhalten*, or variable resistance to PROM), and transcortical motor aphasia (with a dominant hemisphere ACA lesion).

PCA - Deficits can include c/l homonymous hemianopia, c/l hemianesthesia, c/l hemiplegia, c/l hemiataxia, and vertical gaze palsy. *Dominant*-sided lesions can lead to amnesia, color anomia, dyslexia w/o agraphia and simultagnosia (defunct perceptual analysis). *Non-dominant*-sided lesions can lead to prosopagnosia (cannot recognize familiar faces).

The *central post-stroke pain (Dejerine-Roussy or thalamic pain) syndrome* can occur with involvement of the thalamo-geniculate branch. *Weber's syndrome* (penetrating branches to the midbrain) consists of i/l CN III palsy and c/l limb weakness). A b/l PCA stroke can cause the *Anton syndrome* (cortical blindness, with denial) or *Balint's* syndrome, which consists of optic ataxia, loss of voluntary but not reflex eye movements, and an inability to understand visual objects (asimultagnosia).

Brainstem - The *lateral medullary (Wallenberg) syndrome* (PICA) consists of vertigo, nystagmus, dysphagia, dysarthria, dysphonia, i/l Horner's syndrome, i/l facial pain or numbness, i/l limb ataxia, and c/l pain and temp sensory loss. The *"locked-in"* syndrome (basilar artery) is due to b/l pontine infarcts affecting the corticospinal and bulbar tracts, but sparing the reticular activating system. Pts are awake and sensate, but paralyzed and unable to speak. Voluntary blinking and vertical gaze may be intact. The *Anton syndrome* (basilar artery) is cortical blindness with denial.

Lacunar - The more common syndromes include *pure motor hemiplegia*, (post. limb internal capsule [IC]), *pure sensory stroke* (thalamus or parietal white matter), the *dysarthria-clumsy hand syndrome* (basis pontis), and the *hemiparesis-hemiataxia syndrome* (pons, midbrain, IC, or parietal white matter). *"Pseudobulbar palsy"* is caused by ant. IC and corticobulbar pathway lacunes (loss of volitional bulbar motor control, [e.g., dysarthria, dysphagia, dysphonia, face weakness] but involuntary motor control of the same muscles is intact, e.g., can yawn or cough). Emotional lability may be seen.

C. Ischemic Stroke Pharmacotherapy and Intervention

1. Guidelines for acute stroke pharmacotherapy

IV tissue plasminogen activator (tPA) is indicated for acute ischemic stroke w/in 3hrs of symptom onset. Contraindications abound, and its use should be limited to experts in its adminstration[5]. Clinical trials of *IV heparin* in acute ischemic stroke (w/in 12hrs of symptom onset) in *unselected* pt populations are inconclusive[5]. Early anticoagulation is likely to be beneficial in acute cardioembolic and large-artery ischemic strokes, in pts with severe CHF, and for progressing stroke when the suspected mechanism is ongoing thromboembolism[5]. Clinical trials, in general, do *not* show clear benefits for *SC heparin, LMWH, or heparinoids* in the treatment of acute ischemic stroke[5]; but they are recommended for DVT/PE prophylaxis in the absence of contraindications.

Low dose *ASA* (160-325mg) is recommended w/in 48hrs for pts with acute ischemic strokes not receiving thrombolytics or anticoagulation[5]. ASA can be safely used with low-dose SC heparin for DVT prophylaxis.

In general, elevated BPs in the acute period should *not* be aggressively managed unless mean arterial BP (which is (SBP+2DBP)/3) >130 or SBP>220mmHg[6]. The best IV meds appear to be labetalol and enalapril; the best p.o. are captopril and nicardipine[6]. Sublingual Ca channel antagonists should be avoided due to rapid absorption and risk of precipitous secondary declines in BP[6] (with subsequent ischemic events, e.g., MI).

References: **1.** From **Stewart DG**: Stroke rehabilitation: Epidemiologic aspects and acute management. *Arch PMR* 1999;80:S4-7. **2. Roth EJ**: Stroke. In **O'Young BJ**, ed.: *PMR Secrets*, 2nd ed. Hanley & Belfus, 2002. **3.** *Stroke/brain attack reporter's handbook*. National Stroke Association, 1997. **4. Kelly-Hayes M**: Factors influencing survival and need for institutionalization following stroke. *Arch PMR* 1988;69:415-8. **5.** Antithrombotic and thrombolytic therapy for ischemic stroke. In: Sixth American College of Chest Physicians Consensus Conference on Antithrombotic Therapy. *Chest* 2001 Jan;119(1Suppl):300S-20S. **6. Special Writing Group of the AHA Stroke Council**: Guidelines for the management of pts with acute ischemic stroke. *American Heart Association* Pub. No. 71-0054, 1994.

2. Recommendations for secondary prevention

Ongoing lifestyle and medical risk factor modification, such as those identified in the **Framingham Heart Studies** (a series of >1,000 papers originally identifying smoking, HTN, and hypercholesterolemia among others as risk factors for cardiovascular diseases) are warranted.

For *non-cardioembolic* cerebral ischemic events (strokes or TIAs), 1 of the 3 following long-term prophylactic *options* is recommended[1]:

a. *ASA* 50-325mg qd;

b. ASA 25mg bid + extended-release dipyridamole 200mg bid (*Aggrenox*);

c. clopidogrel (*Plavix*) 75mg qd (acceptable for ASA-allergic pts).

The **CAPRIE** (Clopidogrel versus Aspirin in Patients at Risk of Ischemic Events)[2] trial demonstrated that clopidogrel is slightly better than ASA (5.33% vs. 5.83% overall incident rate) in reducing ischemic events (e.g., MI, stroke) in a study of 19,185 pts with known atherosclerotic disease (8.7% risk reduction vs. ASA, p=0.045).

For *cardioembolic* cerebral ischemic events, oral anticoagulation with a target INR of 2.5 (range, 2.0-3.0) is recommended[1]. INRs >3.0 are associated with a higher risk of brain hemorrhage that outweighs the potential benefit[1].

The **NASCET** (North American Symptomatic Carotid Endarterectomy Trial)[3] study demonstrated a 6-10× reduction in long-term risk of stroke following carotid endarterectomy (CEA) versus medical management alone for patients with recent stroke or TIA with extracranial internal carotid artery stenosis of 70-99%. The benefit, however, was largely dependent on the skill of the surgeon. CEA for stenosis <70% was not supported. ASA, 81-325mg qd, is recommended before and after the CEA[1]. Guidelines for incidentally discovered asymptomatic carotid stenosis are less clear.

C. Post-Acute Medical Complications

The major *causes of death* during the 1st month post-stroke, in order of decreasing frequency, are the stroke itself (i.e., progressive cerebral edema and herniation), pneumonia, cardiac disease, and pulmonary embolism[4]. Complications noted during the *post-acute stroke rehabilitation period* include pneumonia and pulmonary aspiration (40%), UTI (40%), musculoskeletal pain/RSD (30%), depression (30%), falls (25%), venous thromboembolism (6%), seizure (4%), and pressure ulcer (3%)[5].

Incidence of *urinary incontinence* is 50-70% during the 1st month post-stroke and about 15% after 6mos (comparable to the general population)[4]. Tx can include timed-voiding, fluid intake regulation, and tx of UTIs.

Glenohumeral subluxation, seen in 30-50% of pts, may play a role in post-stroke shoulder pain[5]. Arm trough or lapboard use while sitting, stretching of the shoulder depressors/internal rotators, and avoiding pulling on the affected arm during transfers can be key aspects of management during the early rehabilitation phase. If spasticity becomes severe, a subscapularis phenol/botulinum toxin injection can sometimes be helpful[5].

Dysphagia in pts with unilateral stroke usually improves rapidly, and by 1 month post-stroke, only ~2% of pts still have difficulty[5]. Pts with brainstem strokes may progress more slowly and require g-tube feeding[5].

D. Motor Recovery Following Stroke

Twitchell gave the first systematic clinical description of motor recovery following stroke[6]. In particular, tone and "stereotypic" movements, characterized by a tight coupling of movement at adjacent joints (later termed "synergy" by Brunnstrom), were noted to develop before isolated voluntary motor control was re-established. In addition, it was noted that motor control returned proximally before distally and LEx fxn recovered earlier and more completely than UEx. Poor prognostic indicators included severe proximal spasticity, proprioceptive facilitation response not present by 9days, onset of movement at >2-4wks, absence of voluntary hand movement at 4-6wks, or a prolonged flaccid period. Full recovery, when it occurred, was usually complete w/in 12wks.

Brunnstrom later formalized the stages of motor recovery[7]:

I   Flaccid limb.

II   Some spasticity with weak flexor and extensor synergies.

III Prominent spasticity; voluntary motion occurs w/in synergy patterns.

IV   Some selective activation of muscles outside of synergy patterns. Spasticity reduced.

V   Most limb movement independent from limb synergy; spasticity further reduced but still present with rapid movements.

VI   Near normal coordination with isolated movements.

VII Restoration to normal.

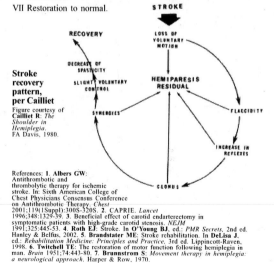

Stroke recovery pattern, per Cailliet

Figure courtesy of **Cailliet R**: *The Shoulder in Hemiplegia.* FA Davis, 1980.

References: **1. Albers GW**: Antithrombotic and thrombolytic therapy for ischemic stroke. In: Sixth American College of Chest Physicians Consensus Conference on Antithrombotic Therapy. *Chest* 2001;119(1Suppl):300S-320S. **2.** CAPRIE. *Lancet* 1996;348:1329-39. **3.** Beneficial effect of carotid endarterectomy in symptomatic patients with high-grade carotid stenosis. *NEJM* 1991;325:445-53. **4. Roth EJ**: Stroke. In **O'Young BJ**, ed.: *PMR Secrets*, 2nd ed. Hanley & Belfus, 2002. **5. Brandstater ME**: Stroke rehabilitation. In **DeLisa J.** ed.: *Rehabilitation Medicine: Principles and Practice,* 3rd ed. Lippincott-Raven, 1998. **6. Twitchell TE**: The restoration of motor function following hemiplegia in man. *Brain* 1951;74:443-80. **7. Brunnstrom S**: *Movement therapy in hemiplegia: a neurological approach.* Harper & Row, 1970.

E. Neurophysiological Therapies

The neurodevelopmental treatment approach (NDT) (Bobath) is widely used in the CNS rehabilitation of infants through adults. Some key concepts include 1) the suppression of abnormal tone, posture, and reflex patterns; 2) the "relearning" of normal movement through facilitating selective automatic responses (often using touch and pressure applied by the therapist); and 3) the adoption of appropriate postures for a given task.

Proprioceptive neuromuscular facilitation (PNF) (Kabat, Voss) is originally based on concepts developed by Kabat in the 1940s for the tx of paralysis, and uses spiral, diagonal patterning techniques to facilitate the proprioceptive system. The term PNF also describes a technique of improving ROM by alternating ~6sec isometric contractions at terminal AROM with passive (aided) stretching beyond that point.

Constraint-induced movement therapy (CIMT) involves restraining the non-hemiplegic (upper) limb to force use of the affected limb. Recent research has shown CIMT is 1) feasible/ tolerated and 2) associated with less short-term arm impairment than traditional therapy[1]. The **Brunnstrom method** uses primitive postural reactions and *synergies* to facilitate motor function. The **Rood method** uses cutaneous stimuli (e.g., brushing, icing) to activate motor function and inhibit spastic antagonists.

Note: Therapists may often utilize aspects of several of the above therapy approaches when formulating a treatment plan for an individual pt.

F. Functional Outcome Following Stroke

It is generally estimated that only ~1 in 10 are functionally independent at the time of stroke and nearly one-half are independent at 6mos[2]. Most improvement in ADLs occurs during the 1st 6mos, although up to 5% of pts may show continued measurable improvement at 12mos post-stroke[3]. Typical frequencies of disabilities in some specific activities at 6mos post-stroke are as follows: unable to walk (15%), needs assist to transfer (20%), needs assist to bathe (50%), and needs assist to dress (30%)[2].

The **Copenhagen Stroke Studies**[4,5] are an extensive, ongoing series of papers with descriptions of stroke rehabilitation outcomes. One recurrent theme is that short-term and long-term morbidity/ mortality and rehabilitation outcome are positively affected by special stroke units (vs. general medical or neurologic units)[4]. Generally, length of hospital stay is also significantly reduced. Another theme is that initial stroke recovery is generally the most important factor in both neurologic and functional recovery. Best neurologic recovery is seen by 11wks for 95% of patients; most ADL recovery (by Barthel Index) is by 12.5wks with daily PT/OT, but recovery could take 2yrs or more[5]. Although the prognosis in patients with mild or moderate stroke is usually excellent, periodic rehabilitation interventions may be necessary to maintain function.

1. Dromerick AW: Does the application of CIMT during acute rehabilitation reduce arm impairment after ischemic stroke? *Stroke* 2000;31:2984-8. **2. Roth EJ:** Stroke. In **O'Young BJ**, ed.: *PMR Secrets,* 2nd ed. Hanley & Belfus, 2002. **3. Brandstater ME:** Stroke rehabilitation. In **DeLisa J**, ed.: *Rehabilitation Medicine: Principles and Practice,* 3rd ed. Lippincott-Raven, 1998. **4. Jorgensen HS:** The effect of a stroke unit: reductions in mortality, discharge rate to nursing homes, length of hospital stay, and cost. *Stroke* 1995;26:1178-82. **5. Jorgensen HS:** Outcome and time course of recovery in stroke. *Arch PMR* 1995;76:406-12.

XVIII. SPINAL CORD INJURY (SCI)

A. Epidemiology of Traumatic SCI

There are ~11,000 new cases in the U.S. who survive each year[1]. Mean age at time of injury is 32.3yrs; median is 27yrs[1]. ♂:♀=4:1. C5 is the most common (15%) neurologic level of injury at time of hospital discharge[2]. 31.1% are incomplete tetraplegics; 27% are complete paraplegics; 21.4% are complete tetraplegics and 20.5% are incomplete paraplegics[1]. U.S. prevalence is expected to be about 250,000 by 2004[2].

According to the Model SCI Care Systems (MSCICS) 1994-1998 data, the most common etiologies are vehicular accidents (40.7%), acts of violence (21.8%), falls (21.3%), and sports (7.9%)[1]. Because the MSCICS (estimated to capture about 13% of all U.S. SCI pts) primarily serves urban areas, acts of violence may be overrepresented in their samples[1].

B. Selected Tracts

The majority of descending *corticospinal fibers* cross at the medulla to become the lateral corticospinal tract (CST). A small number of CST fibers do not decussate at the medulla and descend via the anterior CST before crossing at the level of the anterior white commissure. Although often depicted in many representations of the spinal cord (see below right), the existence of a somatotopic organization of the lateral CST has recently been challenged[3].

The ascending *dorsal white columns* cross in the medulla, via the medial lemniscus, then go on to the thalamus. The *spinothalamic tracts*, which carry pain, temperature, and non-discriminative tactile sensations, cross obliquely in the ventral white commissure of the spinal cord, ascending a level as they do so.

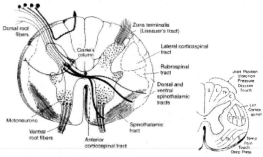

References: **1. Nobunaga AI**: Recent demographic and injury trends in people served by the MSCICS. *Arch PMR* 1999;80:1372-82. **2. Devivo M**: Epidemiology of traumatic SCI. In Kirshblum S. ed.: *Spinal Cord Medicine*. LWW, 2002. **3. Levi AD**: Clinical syndromes associated with disproportionate weakness of the upper versus the lower extremities after cervical spinal cord injury. *Neurosurgery* 1996;38:179-83. Figures courtesy of **Adams M**, ed.: *Adams & Victor's Principles of Neurology*, 7th ed. McGraw-Hill, 2001.

C. Classification of SCI

1. Perform a sensory exam in 28 dermatomes for PP and LT, including rectal sensation. The sensory level is the most caudal level with intact (grade 2) sensation.
2. Perform a supine motor exam of 10 key muscle groups, including voluntary anal contraction. The motor level is the most caudal level with grade ≥3, where all muscles rostral to it are grade 5.
3. Determine the neurologic level, which is the most caudal level at which both sensory and motor modalities are intact bilaterally.
4. Classify as complete or incomplete. Completes have no motor or sensory function, including deep anal sensation, preserved in sacral S4-5. (*Note:* SSEPs may be useful in differentiating complete versus incomplete SCI in pts who are uncooperative or unconscious. SSEPs are also unaffected by spinal shock.)
5. Categorize by American Spinal Injury Association (ASIA) Impairment Scale, A-E. (Determine the zone of partial preservation if ASIA A.)

ASIA key sensory points

C2 Occipital protuberance	T1 Medial antecubital fossa	L3 Medial anterior knee
C3 Supraclavicular fossa	T2 Apex of the axilla	L4 Medial malleolus
C4 Top of the AC joint	T4 Medial to nipple	L5 Medial dorsal foot
C5 Lateral antecubital fossa	T10 Lateral to umbilicus	S1 Inf. lat. malleolus
C6 Dorsal proximal thumb	T12 Inguinal ligament	S2 Popliteal fossa
C7 Dorsal proximal mid finger	L1 B/t T12 and L2	S3 Ischial tuberosity
C8 Dorsal proximal 5th finger	L2 Medial anterior thigh	S4-5 Anal mucocutan jxn

ASIA key muscles

C5 Elbow flexors	T1 Small finger abductors	L5 EHL
C6 Wrist extensors	L2 Hip flexors	S1 Ankle PF
C7 Elbow extensors	L3 Knee extensors	
C8 FDP of 3rd digit	L4 Ankle DF	

Sensory are scored as 0 (absent), 1 (impaired, including hyperaesthesia), 2 (normal), or NT. When scoring PP, inability to distinguish PP from LT is scored 0/2. Muscles are graded from 0 (total paralysis) to 5 (normal active movement with FROM against full resistance), or NT.

ASIA Impairment Scale, Revised (2000)

A Complete - No sensory or motor function is preserved in the sacral segments S4-5. The zone of partial preservation (only used in ASIA A) refers to the most caudal segment with some sensory or motor function.

B Incomplete - Sensory but no motor function is preserved below the neurologic level and includes sacral segments S4-5.

C Incomplete - Motor function is preserved below the neurologic level, and more than half of the key muscles below the neurologic level have a muscle grade <3.

D Incomplete - Motor function is preserved below the neurologic level, and at least half of key muscles below the neurologic level have a muscle grade ≥3.

E Normal - Sensory and motor function are normal.

Note: For an individual to receive a grade of ASIA C or D, there must be sensory or motor S4-5 sparing. In addition, the individual must have either: 1) voluntary anal sphincter contraction or 2) sparing of motor function >3 levels below the motor level.

Reference: **American Spinal Injury Association**: *International Standards for Neurological Classification of SCI, revised 2000, reprinted 2002.* Chicago, IL, ASIA, 2002.

D. Spinal Cord Injury Clinical Syndromes

Anterior cord - These may be due to retropulsed disks/vertebral fragments, aortic clamping during surgery, or lesions of the anterior spinal artery. Intraoperative SSEPs (which primarily monitor the posterior column pathways) may miss the development of an anterior cord syndrome. There is variable loss of motor and pinprick sensation, with relative preservation of proprioception and light touch. Prognosis for motor recovery is generally considered poor.

Brown-Sequard - Etiologies may include stab wounds or tumors. Hemisection of the cord produces ipsilateral weakness, hyperreflexia, and proprioceptive loss and contralateral loss of pinprick and temperature sense. The prognosis for ambulation is best among the incomplete SCI syndromes.

Cauda equina - Cauda equina injuries may be due to neural canal compression or fxs of the pelvis, sacrum, or spine at L2 or below. The syndrome can be described as "multiple radiculopathies" since the cauda is comprised of lumbosacral nerve roots. Sequelae depend on the roots involved and may include bowel/bladder areflexia, erectile dysfunction, saddle anesthesia, and flaccid LEx weakness that can progress to complete paraplegia. Radicular pain is common and can be severe. Anal, bulbocavernosus, plantar, and ankle deep tendon reflexes may be lost. Recovery is possible because the nerve roots can regenerate. Consultation for possible early, but not necessarily emergent, surgery is indicated.

Central cord - This syndrome is typically seen in older persons with cervical spondylosis following neck hyperextension injury, resulting in upper > lower limb involvement and sparing of the lowest sacral segments. Bowel, bladder, and sexual dysfunction is variable. The postulated mechanism of injury involves cord compression both anteriorly and posteriorly, with inward bulging of the ligamentum flavum during hyperextension in a stenotic spinal canal[1]. Penrod retrospectively studied 51 pts with central cord syndrome and noted better overall recovery of ambulation, self-care, and bowel/bladder function in pts <50 yrs of age (n=30) than their older counterparts (n=21) at time of discharge from rehabilitation[2].

Conus medullaris - A pure conus medullaris lesion (e.g., intramedullary tumor) can result in saddle anesthesia and bladder/anal sphincter/erectile dysfunction due to cord injury at S2-4. Anal (S2-4), bulbocavernosus (S2-4), and ankle deep tendon reflexes (S1,S2) may be lost if there is injury to the corresponding level of the spinal cord. Prognosis for recovery is poor.

Conus medullaris lesions due to trauma (e.g., L1 vertebral body fx) are typically accompanied by injury of some of the lumbosacral nerve roots, resulting in a variable degree of LEx dysfunction.

References: **1. Kirshblum S**: Neurologic assessment and classification of traumatic SCI. In **Kirshblum S**, ed.: *Spinal Cord Medicine*. LWW, 2002. **2. Penrod LE**: Age effect on prognosis for functional recovery in acute, traumatic central cord syndrome. *Arch PMR* 1990;71:963-8. Figures courtesy of **American Spinal Injury Association**: *Standards for Neurological and Functional Classification of SCI*, 3rd ed. Chicago, IL, ASIA, 1990.

E. Basis for Acute Interventions

Steroids are thought to be neuroprotective in acute SCI by inhibiting lipid peroxidation and scavenging free radicals. The use of IV methylprednisolone (MP) in acute non-penetrating traumatic SCI is supported by the *National Acute Spinal Cord Injury Studies* (NASCIS)[1,2]. The results of the NASCIS trials, however, have been challenged by some authors[3,4].

In *NASCIS 2*, segmental and long-tract neurologic function were modestly improved at 6wks, 6mos, and 1yr post-SCI in pts receiving MP w/in 8hrs of SCI versus placebo or naloxone. MP was given as a 30mg/kg bolus over 15min, followed by a 45min gap, then as a 5.4mg/kg/hr drip x23hrs. *NASCIS 3* further refined the MP protocol—if initiated w/in 3hrs of SCI, administer MP x24hrs; if initiated 3-8hrs post-SCI, administer x48hrs.

GM-1 ganglioside (Sygen) has demonstrated neuroprotective and neuroregenerative effects *in vitro*. The *Sygen Multicenter Acute SCI Study*[5] showed a more rapid time course of neurologic recovery in the Sygen + IV MP versus the IV MP group, but similar outcomes at 26wks.

The optimal timing for *surgery* after SCI is unknown. Retrospective data suggest a role for urgent decompression in the setting of b/l facet dislocation or incomplete SCI with progressive neurologic deterioration[6].

References: **1. Bracken MB**: NASCIS 2. *NEJM* 1990;322:1405-11. **2. Bracken MB**: NASCIS 3. *JAMA* 1997;277:1597-604. **3. Nesathurai S**: Steroids and SCI: revisiting NASCIS 2 and 3. *J Trauma* 1998;45:1088-93. **4. Hurlbert RJ**: Methylprednisolone for acute SCI: an inappropriate standard of care. *J Neurosurg* 2000;93(1 Suppl):1-7. **5. Geisler F**: Sygen Multicenter study. *Spine* 2001;26(Suppl):87-98. **6. Fehlings MG**: The role and timing of decompression in acute SCI. *Spine* 2001;26(Suppl):101-9.

F. Prognosis and Recovery in Traumatic SCI

Complete SCI - Only 2-3% of pts who are ASIA A at 1wk post-SCI improve to ASIA D by 1yr[1]. In *complete tetraplegia*, >95% of key muscles with grade 1 or 2 at one month post-SCI will reach grade 3 at 1yr[1]. ~25% of the most cephalad grade 0 muscles at 1 month recover to grade 3 at 1yr[1]. Most upper limb recovery occurs during the 1st 6mos, with the greatest rate of recovery during the 1st 3mos. Motor level is superior to the neurologic or sensory level in correlating function. In pts who are *complete paraplegics* at 1wk post-SCI, neurologic level of injury has been found to remain unchanged at 1yr in 73%, improve 1 level in 18%, improve ≥2 levels in 9%[1]. Waters reported that only 5% of complete paraplegics eventually achieve community ambulation[2].

Incomplete SCI - *Incomplete tetraplegics* often recover multiple levels below the initial level. Waters reported that 46% of incomplete tetraplegics recover sufficient motor recovery to ambulate at 1yr[3]. 80% of *incomplete paraplegics* regain hip flexors and knee extensors (grade ≥3) by 1yr[1].

In a review of 27 pts who were initially sensory incomplete, Crozier reported that partial (or greater) preservation of pinprick sensation below the zone of injury was predictive of eventual functional ambulation[4].

Miscellaneous - The 72hr post-SCI neurologic exam may more reliably predict recovery than an exam performed on the day of injury[5]. Absence of the *bulbocavernosus reflex* beyond the first few days can signify a lower motor neuron lesion and have implications on bowel, bladder, and sexual function. On *MRI*, presence of hemorrhage and length of edema are independent negative predictors of motor function at 1yr[1]. Strength ≥3/5 in the b/l HFs and one KE correlate with community ambulation[6].

References: **1. Ditunno JF**: Predicting outcome in traumatic SCI. In **Kirshblum S**, ed.: *Spinal Cord Medicine.* LWW, 2002. **2. Waters RL**: Donald Munro Lecture: Functional and neurologic recovery following acute SCI. *J Spinal Cord Med* 1998;21:195-9. **3. Waters RL**: Motor and sensory recovery following incomplete tetraplegia. *Arch PMR* 1994;75:306-11. **4. Crozier KS**: SCI: Prognosis for ambulation based on sensory examination in pts who are initially motor complete. *Arch PMR* 1991;72:119-21. **5. Maynard FM**: Neurologic prognosis after traumatic quadriplegia: 3-yr experience of California regional SCI care system. *J Neurosurg* 1979;50:611-6. **6. Hussey RW**: SCI: Requirements for ambulation. *Arch PMR* 1973;54:544-7.

G. Expected Functional Levels
(I, independent; A, assist; D, dependent.)

C1-3 - Ventilator-dependent (or may have phrenic nerve pacing); D for secretion management. I with power WC mobility and pressure relief with equipment, otherwise essentially D for all care (but I for directing care).

C4 - May be able to breathe w/o a ventilator. May use a mobile arm support for limited ADLs if there is some elbow flexion and deltoid strength.

C5 - May require A to clear secretions. May be I for feeding after setup and with adaptive equipment, e.g., a long opponens orthosis with utensil slots and mobile arm support. Requires A for most upper body ADLs. Most pts will be *unable* to do self clean intermittent catheterization (CIC). I with power WC; some users may be I with manual WC on non-carpeted, level, indoor surfaces. Some may drive specially adapted vans.

C6 - May use a tenodesis orthosis and short opponens orthosis with utensil slots. I with feeding except for cutting food. I for most upper body ADLs after setup and with modifications (e.g., velcro straps on clothing); A to D for most lower body ADLs, including bowel care. Some males may be I with CIC after setup; females are usually D. Some pts may be I for transfers using a sliding board and heel loops, but many will require A. May be I with manual WC; but power WCs are also often used, especially for longer distances. May drive a specially adapted van.

C7 - Essentially I for most ADLs, often using a short opponens splint and universal cuff. May require A for some lower body ADLs. Women may have difficulty with CIC. Bowel care may be I with adaptive equipment, but suppository insertion may still be difficult. I for mobility at a manual WC level, except for uneven transfers. Pt may be I with a non-van automobile if the pt can transfer and load/unload the WC.

C8 - Completely I with ADLs and mobility using manual WC and car.

Paraplegia - Trunk stability improves with lower lesions. *Upper and mid thoracics* may stand and ambulate with b/l KAFOs and Lofstrand crutches (i.e., swing-through or swing-to gait), but the intent is usually exercise, not mobility. Using orthotics and gait assistive devices, *lower thoracics and L1* SCI pts can do household ambulation and may be I community ambulators. *L2-S5* SCI pts may be community ambulators with or w/o orthotics (i.e., KAFOs or AFOs) and/or gait assistive devices. (AFOs generally compensate for the ankle weakness, while canes and crutches primarily compensate for hip abduction and extension weakness.)

H. Selected Issues in SCI

Autonomic dysreflexia (AD) - It can occur in 48-85% of pts with SCI at T6 or above[1]. (Since resting SBPs can be 90-110mm Hg in this population, SBPs of 20-40mm Hg >baseline may signify AD[1].) A strong sensory impulse below the injury causes reflex sympathetic vasoconstriction (BP ↑). Due to the SCI, higher CNS centers cannot directly ↓ the sympathetic response. The body attempts to ↓ BP by carotid and aortic baroreceptor/vagal-mediated bradycardia, but this is usually ineffective. See p.134 for tx.

Long-term routine urinary tract surveillance after SCI - *Upper tract* f/u can include *renal scan with GFR* or *renal scan with 24hr Cr clearance* qyr to follow renal function. *US* can be done qyr to detect hydronephrosis and nephrolithiasis. *Lower tract* f/u can include *urodynamics* (UDS) once the bladder starts exhibiting uninhibited contractions (or at around 3-6mos post-injury), then as determined by the clinician (often done qyr or q2yr). Routine *cystoscopy* to potentially diagnose neoplasm at an earlier rather than later stage should be performed qyr after 10yrs of chronic indwelling (urethral or suprapubic) catheter use or sooner (after 5yrs) if there are additional risk factors (heavy smoker, age>40, h/o many UTIs).

Posttraumatic syringomyelia - It is seen in ~3-8% of posttraumatic SCI pts as neurologic decline, or up to 20% on autopsy. It can develop as early as 2mos to yrs post-SCI[3]. Pain is often worsened by coughing or straining, but not by lying supine. Ascending sensory loss, progressive weakness (including bulbar muscles), ↑ sweating, orthostasis, and Horner's syndrome may also be seen. Dx is by MRI. Tx is usually observational and symptomatic. Surgical interventions are available for large, progressive lesions.

Sexual function, fertility - *Females*: 44-55% of women with SCI can achieve orgasm[2]. Menses typically returns w/in 6mos post-SCI, and reproductive function is preserved. Incidence of prematurity and small-for-date infants is high, but there is no increase in spontaneous abortions. Spinal anesthesia is recommended during delivery for pts with SCI at T6 or above.

Males: With *complete* SCI, reflexogenic erections can usually be achieved, although ejaculation is rare. With *incomplete* SCI, reflexogenic erections are usually attainable; ejaculation is less rare than for completes; and some pts can achieve psychogenic erections. Complete or incomplete injuries *below T11* may result in erections of poor quality and duration. Infertility is common after SCI, due to factors including retrograde ejaculation and poor sperm quantity and motility. *Electrovibration* for ejaculation (the ventral penile shaft is stimulated) requires that the pt be >6mos post-injury and have L2-S1 intact. *Electroejaculation* (seminal vesicle and prostatic stimulation through the rectum) is another option.

Tendon transfer surgery - Triceps function can be restored in the C5,6 SCI pt with a posterior deltoid-to-triceps or a biceps-to-triceps transfer. Lateral key grip can be restored in a C6 SCI pt via the modified *Moberg procedure*, which involves attachment of the brachioradialis (C5,6) to the flexor pollicis longus (C8,T1) and stabilization of the thumb CMC and IP joints.

References: **1. Campagnolo D**: Autonomic and CV complications of SCI. In **Kirshblum S**, ed.: *Spinal Cord Medicine.* LWW, 2002. **2. Sipski ML**: Sexual arousal and orgasm in women: the effects of SCI. *Ann Neurol* 2001;49:35-44. **3. Little JW**: Neuromusculoskeletal complications of SCI. In **Kirshblum S**, ed.: *Spinal Cord Medicine.* LWW, 2002.

XIX. MISCELLANY

A. Bladder

Neurophysiology - Bladder distention activates detrusor stretch (delta) receptors, which in turn activate the *sacral micturition center* at S2-4. During bladder filling, the intact cerebral cortex inhibits the sacral micturition center and reflex bladder contraction. Also, *sympathetic efferents* (arising from ~T10-L2, hypogastric nerve) stimulate fundal β-receptors (relaxation), and trigonal/bladder neck α-receptors (contraction), the overall effect of which is storage. (Mnemonic: *s*ympathetic is for *s*torage; *p*arasympathetic is for *p*eeing.)

First sensation of bladder filling is typically ~100cc. Fullness may be appreciated at ~300-400cc. Voluntary continence is maintained via *somatic efferents* (Onuf's nucleus, S2-4, pudendal nerve), which innervate the external urethral sphincter.

With voiding, urethral sphincter pressure drops and the detrusor contracts (stimulated by *parasympathetic fibers* from the sacral micturition center, traveling in the pelvic nerves). This synergic interaction between sphincter and detrusor is coordinated by the *pontine micturition center.*

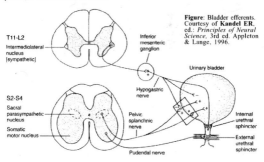

Figure: Bladder efferents. Courtesy of **Kandel ER.** ed.: *Principles of Neural Science,* 3rd ed. Appleton & Lange, 1996.

T11-L2
Intermediolateral nucleus [sympathetic]

S2-S4
Sacral parasympathetic nucleus
Somatic motor nucleus

Inferior mesenteric ganglion

Hypogastric nerve

Pelvic splanchnic nerve

Pudendal nerve

Urinary bladder

Internal urethral sphincter

External urethral sphincter

Neurogenic bladder - A *suprapontine* (i.e., TBI, stroke) lesion can cause detrusor hyperreflexia, w/o detrusor-sphincter dyssynergia (DSD). Symptoms may include frequency and incontinence ("failure to store"). *Tx* options may include timed voids (i.e., offer bedpan q2hrs), urinary collection devices (i.e., condom catheter), or anticholinergics (e.g., oxybutynin).

A *suprasacral* SCI can cause DSD, which is characterized by a lack of sphincter relaxation during bladder contraction. This may manifest as urinary retention ("failure to empty") and eventually result in vesicoureteral reflux due to high bladder contraction pressures. *Tx* options include clean intermittent catheterization (CIC) (e.g., volumes <400-500) + oral or intravesical anticholinergics (e.g., capsaicin, Resinif-Eratoxin), α-adrenergic blockers, indwelling catheterization, stent placement, sphincterotomy, sphincter botulinum injection, or neurostimulation. Potential complications of "cold knife" sphincterotomy include infection, bleeding, strictures, and erectile dysfunction. Laser sphincterotomy complication rates have been relatively favorable. Neurostimulation (e.g., *Vocare System*) provides voiding on demand with low PVRs; it may be used after complete SCI as long as reflex bladder contractions are intact. Bowel programs, however, may be affected (e.g., concomitant BM with voiding, ↓ response to suppositories and digital stimulation).

A *sacral or peripheral nerve lesion* can cause detrusor areflexia, which may manifest as retention or overflow incontinence. *Tx* options may include Valsalva maneuver, suprapubic pressure (Crede) or percussion, cholinergic agonists (e.g., bethanechol), CIC, or indwelling catheter.

B. Deep Venous Thrombosis

1. Selected chemoprophylaxis options

Unfractionated heparin (UH) - UH binds with antithrombin III to inhibit factor IIa (thrombin) and factor Xa (intrinsic clotting pathway).

LMWH - Mechanism of action is similar to UH, but the reduced binding with plasma proteins results in a longer and more predictable half-life. It is contraindicated in heparin-induced thrombocytopenia (HIT)[1]. *Enoxaparin* (Lovenox), 30mg sc bid or 40mg qd, are FDA-approved for s/p TKA. *Dalteparin* (Fragmin), 5000units sc qd, is FDA-approved for s/p THA.

Warfarin[1] - It inhibits the vit.K-mediated production of *pro*coagulant factors X,IX,VII,II (extrinsic pathway) and *anti*coagulant proteins C,S. There is an initial paradoxical procoagulant effect since proteins C,S are depleted first (thus, initiating therapy with "loading" doses >5mg qd is not usually recommended).

For INRs 5-9 w/o significant bleeding, give 1-2.5mg p.o. vit.K or follow INRs w/o vit.K. For INRs >9 w/o significant bleeding, give 3-5mg p.o. vit.K and monitor INRs (repeat vit.K if necessary). For elevated INRs with serious bleeding, give 10mg vit.K by slow IV infusion (repeat q12hrs if nec.) and supplement with plasma or prothrombin complex concentrate.

Other - *Fondaparinux*, 2.5mg sc qd (Arixtra), a heparin-derivative that selectively inhibits factor Xa, is FDA-approved for s/p hip fx, THA, and TKA. *Hirudins* (e.g., Lepirudin, 15mg sc bid) are direct thrombin inhibitors indicated in the setting of HIT. *Heparinoids* (e.g., Danaparoid, no longer available for non-medical reasons) have a similar mechanism of action as UH, but do *not* contain heparin and are also used in the setting of HIT. *ASA* inhibits platelet aggregation, but is *not* recommended by the ACCP for DVT prophylaxis because other measures are more efficacious[1]. *Inferior vena cava filters* are used for PE (*not* DVT) prophylaxis.

2. DVT prophylaxis in selected conditions

Orthopedic surgery - At least 7-10days of LMWH or warfarin (INR 2-3) are recommended *s/p THA, TKA*[1]. Elastic stockings or intermittent pneumatic compression may provide additional efficacy.

LMWH or warfarin (INR 2-3) are also recommended *s/p hip fx surgery*. UH is an alternative option for hip fx surgery pts, but data are limited.

Medical/neuro pts - Low dose sc UH (e.g., 5000units bid) or LMWH are recommended for pts with general medical issues (e.g., cancer, bedrest) or following *ischemic stroke* with impaired mobility[1]. The ideal time to start anticoagulation (AC) after hemorrhagic stroke has not been determined.

SCI[2] - Mechanical and AC tx should be initiated as early as possible provided there is no active bleeding or coagulopathy. Compression hose and boots should be applied for 2wks (r/o DVT first if thromboprophylaxis has been delayed >72 hrs).

For *ASIA A,B* - UH adjusted to high normal aPTT or LMWH for ≥8 wks. For *ASIA A,B with other risk factor(s)* (e.g., LEx, cancer, previous thrombosis, heart failure, obesity, age >70) - UH adjusted to high normal aPTT or LMWH for 12wks or d/c from rehabilitation. *ASIA C* - UH, 5000units q12h, or LMWH for up to 8wks. *ASIA D* - UH, 5000units q12h, or LMWH while in hospital.

3. DVT treatment

In the absence of contraindications, initial tx is typically *IV heparin*. *Warfarin* is usually started w/in 24hrs of DVT dx, once the heparin is therapeutic. A 5mg initial dose of warfarin is preferred over a dose of 10mg due to early paradoxic hypercoagulability. Heparin is d/c'ed when the INR has been ≥2 for 2 consecutive days. Warfarin is typically instituted for 3-6mos.

LMWH (e.g., enoxaparin, 1mg/kg sc bid, or dalteparin, 200units/ kg sc qd) + warfarin is an alternative for the oupt tx of uncomplicated DVT; LMWH can be d/c'ed after 5days and INR>2[3]. *Thrombolytics* may have a role in pts with extensive proximal DVT and low bleed risk. The tx of isolated calf DVT remains controversial.

References: **1**. Prevention of venous thromboembolism. In: 6th American College of Chest Physicians Consensus Conference on Antithrombotic Tx. *Chest* 2001;119(1Suppl):132S-75S. **2**. *Clinical Practice Guideline: Thromboembolism*, 2nd ed. Consortium for Spinal Cord Medicine, 1999. **3. Levine M**: A comparison of home LMWH vs. hospital UH for proximal DVT. *NEJM* 1996;334:677-81.

C. Heterotopic Ossification (HO)

Introduction - HO is the formation of bone in soft tissue, due to the metaplasia of mesenchymal cells into osteoblasts. HO is typically seen near large joints and below levels of neurologic injury. If HO is suspected, a plain x-ray or bone scan may be obtained. The bone scan may be positive at least one wk before x-ray; phases 1 and 2 of the bone scan are highly sensitive. The differential dx can include DVT, septic arthritis, cellulitis, osteomyelitis, hematoma, hemarthrosis, or CRPS.

Reports of incidence in the literature vary, depending on methodology used and whether clinically silent HO is included. In *burns*, common sites include elbow (posterior>anterior) > shoulder (adult) or hip (children). HO location may not coincide with the area of the burn. In *SCI*, HO is seen at the hip (anterior>posterior) > knee > shoulder > elbow. With *TBI*, UEx equals LEx; shoulder ≃ elbow ≃ hip. Hip HO is commonly seen following *THA*. HO may occur at the distal end of *amputated limbs*.

Tx - *Rest* of the acutely involved joint for ≤2wks is acceptable to ↓ inflammation and microscopic hemorrhages[1]. *Ice* may also be helpful. *ROM exercises* are controversial, although *gentle*, painless PROM or AROM is usually recommended. More aggressive ROM may be initiated after the first 2wks, but must be curtailed if erythema or swelling increases[1]. Immobilization in a functional position is prudent if ankylosis is inevitable.

Medical options include NSAIDs (e.g., *indomethacin*, 25mg po tid x ≥6 wks) or *etidronate* (e.g., 20mg/kg po qd x2wks, then 10mg/kg po qd x 10wks; other regimens exist). Etidronate is thought to reduce further HO formation by reducing osteoblastic/clastic activity and calcium phosphate precipitation[1]. It does *not*, however, treat HO that has already formed.

Surgical resection may be indicated to address significant functional limitations, but only after the HO has matured (determined by a negative 3-phase bone scan and arrested HO formation on serial x-rays). Serum alkaline phosphatase also tends to normalize with maturity. Gentle, early (w/in 48hrs) post-operative ROM is recommended[1].

Reference: **1. Subbarao J**: HO. In **O'Young BJ**, ed.: *PMR Secrets*, 2nd ed. Hanley & Belfus, 2002.

D. Inflammatory Demyelinating Polyneuropathy[1]

Acute inflammatory demyelinating polyradiculoneuropathy (AIDP, Gullain-Barré syndrome) - AIDP is an acquired disease of unknown etiology characterized by ascending parasthesias and weakness that can progress to total body paralysis, autonomic disturbances, and respiratory failure. Global incidence is about 0.4-1.7/100,000; a mild flu-like illness precedes ~60% of cases. >50% of patients will complain of muscular pain and aching. Extraocular muscles and sphincter function are typically spared. Dx is supported by areflexia, progressive weakness in all limbs, relative symmetry of involvement, CSF cytoalbuminologic dissociation (elevated protein, <10 mononuclear cells/mm³) and EDx findings (see p.85).

Plasmapheresis or *IV Ig* (400mg/kg/d x5d) given during the evolution of symptoms (w/in 2wks of onset) are effective and proven to decrease overall recovery time. Glucocorticoids are *not* effective. Early rehabilitation should emphasize *stretching* and *gradual strengthening*; aggressive therapies may cause overwork weakness. A *tilt table* may be useful in patients with autonomic instability. Prescription of appropriate assistive mobility devices and lower limb orthotics is often indicated.

Mortality is about 3-5%, usually due to respiratory or cardio-vascular causes. The majority of patients recover completely or nearly completely. Recovery time can be weeks to months, or up to 6-18mo if axonal damage has occurred. About 10% have a pronounced residual disability, most often lower leg weakness and numbness of the feet. ~5-10% may suffer one or more recurrences of acute polyneuropathy and some cases may evolve into a chronic, progressive inflammatory polyneuropathy.

Chronic inflammatory demyelinating polyradiculoneuropathy - CIDP is similar pathologically to AIDP, but tends to have a slower onset (i.e., over months) and better response to corticosteroids (usual regimen is 80mg prednisone qd, tapered over months to the lowest effective dose).

Reference: **1. Victor M**: *Adams & Victor's Principles of Neurology*, 7th ed. McGraw Hill, 2001.

E. Multiple Sclerosis (MS)

Introduction and epidemiology[1] - MS is a CNS inflammatory disease of unknown etiology (thought to be autoimmune) that is characterized by areas of demyelination that are disseminated in time and space. U.S. prevalence is ~250,000-350,000. The incidence is ~8,800 new cases dx'ed annually with ♀:♂=2:1 and Caucasian>Asian>African-American. Mean onset age is ~30yrs. Incidence and death rates are higher in the northern latitudes; an important factor appears to be where one lives prior to 15yrs of age.

Dx and clinical features - *Definite MS* has been classically defined as ≥2 attacks, separated by ≥1 month, with clinical, imaging, or laboratory evidence (e.g., ↑ CSF protein with oligoclonal bands on electrophoresis, delayed VEP/SSEP latencies) of ≥2 lesions[2]. Each attack should last >24hrs. Ovoid plaques that are bright on T2 MRI are typically found in the periventricular white matter, cortical-subcortical junction, brainstem, and/or cerebellum. Corpus callosum lesions are relatively specific for MS.

Common *presenting symptoms* include sensory changes, visual loss, motor changes, and diplopia. Common *clinical features* include parasthesias, weakness, spasticity, fatigue (may be worsened by heat = Uhthoff's phenomenon), bladder and sexual dysfunction, cognitive changes, depression, dysphagia, and neuropathic pain. Exacerbations are fewer during pregnancy but increased post-partum; fertility is unaffected. *Prognosis* is worse for males, older age of onset, high lesion burden on MRI at onset, initially polysymptomatic, predominantly cerebellar or motor symptoms, and rapidly progressive symptoms.

Clinical categories and tx - *Relapsing-remitting* MS is characterized by acute attacks (<1/month) followed by recovery (w/in wks to mos) with little or no residual neurologic deficit. Interferon β-1a (Avonex, Rebif), interferon β-1b (Betaseron), and glatimer acetate (Copaxone) are effective therapies. Half will develop a *secondary progressive* course with or w/o relapses. Interferon β-1b may delay progression of disability in secondary progressive MS (i.e., WC dependence). These two types comprise ~85% of persons with MS.

Primary progressive MS (10-15%) is characterized by an insidious onset and gradual progression w/o acute relapses. It is typically seen in the elderly; males and females are equally affected. No proven pharmacotherapy assists in tx.

Progressive relapsing MS (<5%) is a progressive disease from the onset with superimposed acute relapses with or w/o some recovery.

IV steroids, which are a mainstay of acute tx (e.g., methylpredniso-lone IV 500mg qd x5d or 1gm qd x3d), shorten the exacerbation period, but do *not* change the ultimate extent of recovery. *Rehabilita-tion* management includes tx of bowel/bladder spasticity and pain issues. Fatigue can be addressed with energy conservation techniques and/or pharmaceuticals (e.g., amantadine, pemoline, modafinil). Exercise, once considered contraindicated in MS, should be prescribed to help delay secondary disability.

References: **1. Anderson DW**: Revised estimate of MS prevalence in the U.S. *Ann Neurol* 1992;31:331-6. **2. Poser CM**: New diagnostic criteria for MS. *Ann Neurol* 1983;13:227-31. **3. Petajan JH**: Impact of aerobic training on fitness and quality of life in MS. *Ann Neurol* 1996;39:432-41. **4. Rudick R**: Management of MS. *NEJM* 1997;337:1604-17.

F. Osteoporosis (OP)

The *WHO definition of OP* is a T-score >2.5 standard deviations below the mean bone mineral denisty (BMD) value for young, healthy, Caucasian women[1]. Predictors of ↓BMD include ♀ gender, Caucasian race, +fam hx, smoking, h/o prior fx, ↑age, and ↓estrogen, weight, or body mass index[1]. EtOH and caffeine are inconsistently associated with ↓BMD[1]. 2° causes of OP include disuse, hyperthyroidism, steroids, and heparin. Muscle pull is more important than weight bearing in disuse OP prevention[2].

1. Supplements and pharmacotherapy

The National Osteoporosis Foundation (NOF) guidelines recommend a *calcium* intake of ≥1200mg/d for all patients (including supplements if nec.), and 400-800 IU/d of *vit. D*[3]. The NOF recommends pharmacotherapy in ♀ with a T-score<-2 in the absence of OP risk factors or a T-score<-1.5 with risk factors[3]. High-risk pts w/ o BMD testing may also be treated.

Estrogen is effective in studies with BMD and vertebral fxs as the primary outcome[1]. Hip fx risk is reduced in observational studies[1]. A *biphosphonate* (e.g., alendronate, risedronate) is recommended if HRT fails or is contraindicated/refused: there is a dose-dependent increase in spine and hip BMD; vertebral fx risk is reduced by 30-50%[1]. The goal of *selective estrogen receptor modulators* (raloxifene) is to maximize the beneficial effect of estrogen on bone while minimizing the deleterious effects on breast and endometrium. Raloxifene has reduced vertebral fx risk by 36% in large clinical trials[1]. *Salmon calcitonin* (100 IU IM/sq qd) improves BMD and reduces vertebral fx risk at the lumbar spine, but not at the hip[1]. Nasal calcitonin (200 IU qd) has similar benefits, but is not as effective in treating bone pain as the injectable[1].

2. Exercise and rehabilitation

The NOF recommends an exercise prevention program, emphasizing weight bearing, of 45-60min/d 4×/wk[3]. Interventions to reduce the risk and/or impact of falls (e.g., appropriate assistive mobility devices, exercise programs, hip padding, avoidance of medications affecting the CNS) may reduce hip fx incidence. Poor back extensor strength correlates with a higher incidence of vertebral fxs[4].

Acute vertebral fxs can be painful and are often managed with *bed rest, orthotic immobilization,* and *analgesics* (e.g., narcotics). NSAIDs should be used with caution. Spine surgery is reserved for rare cases involving neurologic deficits or an unstable spine. Vertebral injection of polymethyl-methacrylate (i.e., *vertebroplasty*) anecdotally improves acute pain; it is unknown, however, if this rigid vertebral reinforcement increases long-term risk of fx of adjacent vertebrae[1]. *Postural training, back extensor exercises, pectoral stretching, walking,* or other weight-bearing exercises are keys to rehabilitation. Rigid orthoses to limit spinal flexion (e.g., CASH, Jewett) may reduce the risk of additional vertebral body fxs.

References: 1. Osteoporosis Prevention, Diagnosis, and Therapy. *NIH Consensus Statement March 27-29,* 2000;17:1-36. 2. **Abramson AS**: Influence of wt-bearing and muscle contraction in disuse OP. *Arch PMR* 1961;42:147-51. 3. *NOF guidelines.* Excerpta Medica, Inc., 1999. 4. Sinaki M: Can strong back extensors prevent vertebral fractures in women with osteoporosis? *Mayo Clin Proc* 1996;71:951-6.

G. Spasticity

Spasticity is a disorder characterized by a velocity-dependent increased resistance to passive stretch, associated with exaggerated tendon jerks, resulting from hyperexcitability of the stretch reflex. Spasticity is part of the *UMN syndrome*, which includes the *positive* symptoms of spasticity and uninhibited flexor reflexes in the lower limbs and the *negative* symptoms of weakness and poor dexterity. Commonly used clinical scales include the modified Ashworth scale and spasm frequency score:

Modified Ashworth Scale[1] score[*2]

0 No increase in tone.
1 Slightly increased tone, with a catch/release or minimal resistance at terminal ROM.
1+ Slightly increased tone, with a catch, followed by minimal resistance throughout the remainder (less than half) of the ROM.
2 Increased tone through most of the ROM, but affected part easily moved.
3 Considerably increased tone; passive movement difficult.
4 Affected part rigid in flexion or extension.

Spasm frequency

0 No spasms
1 Spasms induced by stimulation
2 Infrequent spontaneous spasms (<1/hr)
3 Spontaneous spasms (>1/hr)
4 Spontaneous spasms (>10/hr)
* - by subject self report

Tx

Indications for treating spasticity include pain, decreased function, poor hygiene, skin breakdown, poor cosmesis, and poor positioning. Potential factors that may be exacerbating spasticity (e.g., pressure ulcers, UTIs, bowel impaction, ingrown toenails, SSRIs) should be addressed. Care should be taken before treating any spasticity that may be utilized functionally (e.g., hypertonia in the lower limbs assisting transfers or gait). One algorithm for treating spasticity may be as per the figure at right[1].

References: 1. **Bohannon RW**: Interrater reliability on a modified Ashworth scale of muscle spasticity. *Phys Ther* 1987;67:206-7. 2. **Penn RD**: Intrathecal baclofen for severe spasticity. *Ann NY Acad Sci* 1988;531:15-66. Figure courtesy of **Katz R**: Spasticity. In **O'Young BJ**, ed.: *PMR Secrets*, 2nd ed. Hanley & Belfus, 2002.

110

1. Physical modalities

A *stretching program* should be the cornerstone for most spasticity tx programs. *Splints, casting,* or *bracing* can help preserve ROM by "resetting the muscle spindles." Contractures can be reduced by serially casting a joint (i.e., increasing the stretch stepwise for 1-2 days at a time), although this technique is not always well-tolerated and may lead to skin breakdown. *Cryotherapy* (>15min) may be helpful transiently by reducing the hyperexcitability of the muscle stretch reflex and reducing nerve conduction velocities. *Functional electrical stimulation* (>15min) can improve function and reduce tone for hours after the stimulation (thought to be due to neurotransmitter modulation at the spinal cord level).

2. Pharmaceutical options

Oral medications - These may be indicated for *non-focal* spasticity. Efficacy is often limited by side effects. Options include baclofen, diazepam, dantrolene, clonidine, and tizanidine (see pp.127-33 for details on individual medications). Recently, *gabapentin* showed promising results in the tx of spasticity in a small group of MS pts undergoing a crossover study[1].

Botulinum toxin (BTX) - BTX irreversibly blocks NMJ transmission by inhibiting presynaptic ACh release. BTX-A (Botox, Allergan) is FDA-approved for blepharospasm, strabismus, and cervical dystonia and most recently for severe glabellar (between the eyebrows) frown lines. It is also widely used for spasticity and myofascial pain with favorable results. Onset of effect is typically 24-72 hrs. Peak effect is at 2-6 wks. Clinical efficacy is typically up to 3-4 mos. Recovery is due to axon sprouting.

The theoretical parenteral LD_{50} for a 75kg adult is 3000 units; the recommended maximum dose is 10 units/kg IM (up to 400 units) per visit. At least 3mos between sessions is recommended to decrease the potential for antibody formation. BTX-A is contraindicated in pregnancy, lactation, NMJ disease, and concomitant aminoglycoside use and with human albumin USP allergy. BTX-A should be stored at -5 to -20°C, and should be reconstituted with 0.9% preservative-free saline only. It is available for use for up to 4hrs if refrigerated (2-8°C).

Advantages of BTX-A over phenol include ready diffusion into the injected area (~up to 3-4cm), making injections technically easier, and the absence of dysesthesias (since it is selective for the NMJ).

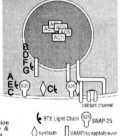

Right: There are 7 distinct BTX subtypes. The BTX heavy chain binds to the presynaptic endplate and the receptor-BTX complex is internalized by endocytosis. The light chain of BTX-A lyses SNAP-25, a protein needed for fusion of ACh vesicles with the presynaptic membrane.

calcium channel

🔌 BTX Light Chain   (S25) SNAP-25

◇ syntaxin   ▯ VAMP/synaptobrevin

Reference: **1**. Cutter NC: Gabapentin effect on spasticity in MS: a placebo-controlled, randomized trial. *Arch PMR* 2000;81:164-9. Figure copyrighted 1997 by John Wiley & Sons, Inc. Adapted and reprinted with permission of Wiley-Liss, Inc., a subsidiary of John Wiley & Sons, Inc. from Spasticity: etiology, evaluation, management, and the role of BTX-A. *Muscle Nerve* 1997;6(Suppl):S151.

Suggested BTX-A adult dosing[1] (in units)

Clinical pattern	Potential muscles involved	Avg starting dose	Range, per visit	# of injection sites
Adducted/internally rotated shoulder	pectoralis complex	100	75-100	4
	latissimus dorsi	100	50-150	4
	teres major	50	25-75	1
	subscapularis	50	25-75	1
Flexed elbow	brachioradialis	50	25-75	1
	biceps	100	50-200	4
	brachialis	50	25-75	2
Pronated forearm	pronator quadratus	25	10-50	1
	pronator teres	40	25-75	1
Flexed wrist	flexor carpi radialis	50	25-100	2
	flexor carpi ulnaris	40	10-50	2
Thumb-in-palm	flexor pollicis longus	15	5-25	1
	adductor pollicis	10	5-25	1
	opponens pollicis	10	5-25	1
Clenched fist	flexor digitorum superficialis	50	25-75	4
	flexor digitorum profundus	15	25-100	2
Intrinsic plus hand	lumbricales interossei	15	10-50/hand	3
Flexed hip	iliacus	100	50-150	2
	psoas	100	50-200	2
	rectus femoris	100	75-200	3
Flexed knee	medial hamstrings	100	50-150	3
	gastrocnemius	150	50-150	4
	lateral hamstrings	100	100-200	3
Adducted thighs	adductor brev/long/magnus	200/leg	75-300	6/leg
Extended knee	quadriceps femoris	100	50-200	4
Equinovarus foot	gastrocnemius medial/lateral	100	50-200	4
	soleus	75	50-100	2
	tibialis posterior	50	50-200	2
	tibialis anterior	75	50-150	3
	flexor digitorum long/brevis	75	50-100	4
	flexor hallucis longus	50	25-75	2
Striatal toe	extensor hallucis longus	50	20-100	2
Neck	sternocleidomastoid*	40	15-75	2
	scalenus complex	30	15-50	3
	trapezius	60	50-150	3
	levator scapulae	80	25-100	3

*The dose should be reduced by half if both SCMs are being injected. **Dosing guidelines**: The recommended maximum dose per visit is 10units/kg, not to exceed 400units. The maximum dose per injection site is 50units. The maximum volume per site is typically 0.5mL. Reinjection should occur no more frequently than q3mos. Consider lowering the dosing if pt's Ashworth scores are in the low range, if pt weight or muscle bulk are low, or if the likely duration of treatment is chronic. Reference: **1.** Table copyrighted 1997 by John Wiley & Sons, Inc. Adapted and reprinted with permission of Wiley-Liss, Inc., a subsidiary of John Wiley & Sons, Inc., from **Brin MF**: Dosing, administration, and a treatment algorithm for use of BTX-A for adult-onset spasticity. *Muscle Nerve* 1997;6(Suppl):S214.

BTX-B (Myobloc) - BTX-B was FDA-approved in 2000 for cervical dystonia. Clinically, it is used for similar indications as BTX-A, although the units are markedly different (initially, 2500-5000 units of BTX-B divided into the affected muscles). BTX-B may be effective in pts who have developed resistance to BTX-A due to repeated use. It may be stored at room temperature for up to 9mos, or 21 mos if refrigerated (2-8°C). It does not need to be reconstituted, but may be diluted with normal saline, in which case it must be used w/in 4hrs.

Phenol (carboxylic acid) - Phenol destroys nerves in a dose-dependent manner, with onset w/in 1hr and a duration that can last years (duration varies widely in the literature). Target nerves are localized with a nerve stimulator and destroyed by direct perineural injection (with subsequent Wallerian degeneration). Alternatively, the motor-point area (located by nerve stimulator) can be injected (e.g., 1-10mL of 3-5% solution IM; max: 10mL of 5%). Recovery with either option occurs by nerve fiber regeneration.

Phenol injections can be combined with BTX injections during a single session, which may be especially useful when there are BTX dosage concerns (i.e., phenol for large, proximal muscles and BTX for smaller, distal muscles). Advantages over BTX include low cost, lack of antibody formation, and longer duration of effect. Disadvantages versus BTX include the greater technical skill involved and potential for dysesthesias, although the latter can be reduced by limiting injections to relatively accessible motor branches of nerves (e.g., pectoral, musculocutaneous, obturator, inferior gluteal, and branches to hamstrings, gastroc-soleus, and tibialis anterior) and avoiding mixed nerve injections (main tibial or median n.). A trial with a local anesthetic (e.g., marcaine 0.25-0.5%) prior to phenol neurolysis can be helpful in predicting the potential effects.

Intrathecal Baclofen (ITB) - ITB is indicated for severe spasticity (Ashworth ≥3) 2° to SCI (FDA-approved in 1992) and severe spasticity of cerebral origin (FDA-approved in 1996). It is also used with fair to good success off-label for severe muscle spasms in chronic back pain and radicular pain. Pts should have a history of poor response to conservative txs and be >4 yrs of age or adequate body wt (>40lbs). A trial of epidural baclofen or a subarachnoid catheter with external pump is often given before implantation of an internal pump. A screening trial of epidural baclofen might be as follows: 50mg epidural bolus on day 1; if not efficacious, 75mg on day 2; if prior doses not successful, 100mg on day 3. A drop in spasticity of ~2 Ashworth grades during the trial may roughly predict efficacy of the implanted pump.

The pump is typically placed in the LLQ to be away from the appendix. The pump is typically refilled q4-12wks (requires a committed patient), and the battery lasts about 5yrs (the pump must be removed to replace the battery). Advantages of ITB include reduced CNS side effects (e.g., sedations) versus oral medications. Potential problems with the implanted system include infection, catheter kinking or dislodgment, and headaches 2° to CSF leak out of the catheter site. The average infusion rate for a lumbar pump is 600 µg/day. Increased spasticity should be worked up and treated before adjusting the ITB dose.

3. Surgical options

Numerous procedures exist, including tendon transfer, tendon/muscle lengthening, and neurosurgical (brain/spinal cord) lesioning. The *split anterior tibial tendon transfer (SPLATT)* (right) procedure can be an effective tx for the spastic equinovarus foot. The lateral portion of the split distal anterior tibialis tendon is reattached to the 3rd cuneiform and cuboid bones. *Achilles tendon lengthening* usually accompanies the SPLATT.

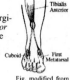

Fig. modified from
Keenan MA:
*Manual of Ortho-
pedic Surgery for
Spasticity.* Raven
Press, 1993.

Selective dorsal rhizotomy may be of some benefit in CP. The procedure involves laminectomy and exposure of the cauda equina. The dorsal rootlets are stimulated individually, and rootlets that produce abnormal EMG responses in limb musculature (believed to be contributing to spasticity) are then severed. Anterior rootlet lesions are undesirable as denervation atrophy may follow, with resultant skin breakdown. Favorable selection criteria for rhizotomy include spastic CP (w/o athetosis), age between 3-8yrs, h/o prematurity, good truncal balance, and a supportive family.

H. Speech & Swallowing

1. Aphasia

Broca's, Wernicke's and global aphasias are the most common. Many cases do *not* fit all the features of the classic syndrome descriptions. The **cortical aphasias** (listed below) usually involve the dominant hemisphere and will have anomia. **Anomic aphasia** (temporal-parietal area, angular gyrus) is poor naming only. **Sub-cortical aphasias** can involve the internal capsule and putamen and are characterized by sparse output and impaired articulation.

Aphasia syndromes (lesion site)	Fluency	Comprehension	Repetition
Global (MCA stem, multilobar)	poor	poor	poor
Transcortical mixed (ACA/PCA watershed areas)	poor	poor	good
Broca's (sup.div. of MCA, Brodmann's areas 44,45 in the prefrontal gyrus)	poor	good	poor
Wernicke's (inf.div. of MCA, Brodmann's areas 21,42 in the posterior, superior temporal gyrus)	good	poor	poor
Transcortical motor (ACA, prefrontal lobe near Broca's area)	poor	good	good
Transcortical sensory (watershed areas, parietooccipital cortex near Wernicke's area)	good	poor	good
Conduction (MCA, arcuate fasciculus)	good	good	poor

Tx of aphasia is individualized to take advantage of residual/recovering function and compensate for deficits, which can vary considerably, even for pts with the same aphasia syndrome. *Melodic intonation therapy* (thought to utilize "musical" areas in the non-dominant hemisphere) may be helpful for pts with expressive aphasia. Family members should be trained to encourage participation of the aphasic pt in conversation and to allow plenty of time for the pt to regain expression.

2. Apraxia and dysarthria

Apraxia of speech is an impairment in the production of syllables and words due to abnormalities in the motor planning of speech, in the *absence* of weakness. Difficulty with polysyllabic words and inconsistency of the phonemic error are typical, e.g., "*bopishmarter*, I mean *doppingor* (supermarket)." Tx consists of intensive speech drills. *Melodic intonation therapy* (utilizing non-dominant hemispheric musical areas) may be helpful for pts with concomitant expressive, but not receptive, aphasia.

Flaccid dysarthria can be the result of weakness of the muscles of articulation (i.e., brainstem or cranial n. pathology). It is character-ized by a breathy, hypernasal, weak voice with imprecise consonant formation. **Ataxic dysarthria** is due to cerebellar disease and is characterized by a slow, slurred, and monopitch voice with an unnatural separation between syllables. **Spastic dysarthria** is due to a UMN lesion and is characterized by a voice that is strained, harsh, hypernasal, and low in pitch and loudness. Speech is slow and characterized by poor prosody.

The essentials of a typical *dysarthria tx* plan are to train the pt to 1) strengthen/coordinate orolingual musculature; 2) slow down the rate of speech; 3) enunciate clearly or "overarticulate"; and 4) become aware of and practice speech at an appropriate loudness.

3. Dysphagia treatment

Suboptimal cognitive status - Feedings should be supervised. For *impulsivity*, present foods one at a time. For *poor judgment*, use small-bowled utensils, covered cups with small openings, and intermittently pinch straws closed to control drinking rate. For *poor attention*, feed in a quiet, distraction-free environment.

Oral phase dysphagia - For *facial weakness*, modify food texture and place food at the back of mouth or on the stronger side, tilt the head toward the stronger side). EMG biofeedback or sucking/blowing exercises may be helpful. For *poor lingual control*, tongue AROM and strengthening can be prescribed (precise articulation should be encouraged).

Pharyngeal phase dysphagia - This is the most common and is often accompanied by a wet, gargly voice with coughing. (Note that an absent gag reflex does not necessarily connote an unsafe swallow; conversely, those with intact gags may aspirate.) Techniques for a *delayed swallow reflex* include chin tuck, head rotation to the weaker side, supraglottic swallow, and thickened liquids. The *chin tuck* maneuver widens the vallecula (allowing the bolus to rest there while the reflex is triggered), reduces the airway opening, and reduces the space between tongue base and posterior pharyngeal wall (increasing pharyngeal pressure). In the *supraglottic swallow*, the pt holds a deep breath with a concomitant Valsalva, swallows, clears the throat, then swallows again, before resuming breathing. Chin tuck and supraglottic swallow are also useful for *reduced laryngeal closure*.

The Mendelsohn maneuver can address *incomplete relaxation or premature closing of the cricopharyngeus*. The pt improves pharyngeal clearance by "holding" a swallow midway for 3-5sec (allowing more complete cricopharyngeal relaxation) before completing the swallow.

XX. Diagnostic Imaging

A. Selected Plain Film Studies

C-spine - On *lateral* view, the anterior vertebral, posterior vertebral, and spinolaminar lines should be aligned. The latter two lines represent the borders of the spinal canal. The intervertebral spaces should be uniform. Prevertebral soft tissues anterior to C2 should not exceed ~30% of the corresponding vertebral body (~50% at C4 and ~100% below C4). Prevertebral swelling may be a sign of bony injury. A Torg ratio of <0.8 is sensitive, but not specific, for spinal stenosis, particularly for persons with larger body mass[1].

Lateral *flexion/extension* views may be helpful in discovering ligamentous injury not apparent on neutral view, but are contraindicated with altered states of consciousness or documented neurologic deficits when being considered as part of an initial trauma evaluation. These views are also useful in assessing stability of a healing post-operative spine.

On *AP* view, the spinous processes should be in line. On *open mouth AP*, the space on either side of the odontoid process should be equal (although rotation may disrupt this). The lateral borders of C1 and C2 should align.

Above: Unilateral facet dislocation, with a disrupted spinous process line.

L-spine - On *lateral* view, the vertebral bodies should be of similar height. The spinous processes should have similar angulations. Decreased intervertebral spaces are suggestive of disk degeneration. Osteophytes may be noted around the edges of the vertebral bodies and facet joints. Vertebral body translation (spondylolisthesis, spinal instability) may sometimes only be noted on flexion/extension views.

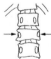

On *AP* view, interpedicular distances should progressively increase from L1 to L5 (note the increase in the L2 interpedicular space vs. L3 in the figure to the left, representing an L2 compression fx).

An *oblique* view (see right) may demonstrate pars interarticularis fxs (a "broken neck" of the "Scotty dog"). The eye of the Scotty dog represents the pedicle; nose = transverse process; ear = superior articular process; foreleg = inferior articular process; body = lamina.

Reference: 1. **Herzog RJ**: Normal cervical morphometry and cervical spinal stenosis in asymptomatic professional football players: plain film radiography, multiplanar CT, and MRI. *Spine* 1991;16:S178-86.

Shoulder - A routine *AP* view with slight humeral external rotation may help to demonstrate arthritic changes and alignment. Wrist weights may be used to test AC ligamentous integrity (the acromion and clavicle should be aligned, and the gap should be <10mm).

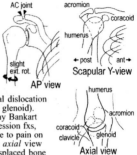

A *scapular Y-view* is easy to obtain and helpful to r/o humeral dislocation (the humerus should overlie the glenoid).

An *axial* view may show bony Bankart lesions and humeral head compression fxs, but may be difficult to obtain due to pain on shoulder abduction. An *oblique axial* view helps detect glenoid fxs with displaced bone and superior humeral head fxs.

Elbow - *AP* and *lateral* views are standard. On the lateral view, a small area of lucency anterior and juxtaposed to the distal humerus represents a fat pad and is a normal finding. An elbow effusion will displace the anterior fat pad further anteriorly and will also make the posterior fat pad visible, which is always an abnormal finding.

Wrist - PA, oblique, and lateral views are the usual basic studies. On *PA*, the proximal and distal margins of the scaphoid, lunate and triquetrum should form smooth curves. *Oblique* views are useful in examining some of the carpal bones, which tend to overlap on PA. A special *scaphoid* view may sometimes be necessary to view scaphoid fxs.

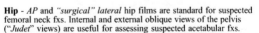

The *lateral* view is useful in assessing the integrity of the radial-lunate-capitate-metacarpal articulations. The "spilled teacup" sign (see left), for instance, indicates lunate dislocation.

Hip - *AP* and *"surgical" lateral* hip films are standard for suspected femoral neck fxs. Internal and external oblique views of the pelvis (*"Judet"* views) are useful for assessing suspected acetabular fxs.

Loosening of the femoral component of a hip prosthesis is supported by a linear lucency >2mm or any progressive lucency. A post-contrast view demonstrating contrast seepage between metal and cement is confirmatory. Acetabular component loosening is supported by a change in position of the component by >4° or 4mm.

Knee - An initial trauma set includes *AP*, *lateral* and *oblique* views. Severe ligamentous or meniscal injuries are usually accompanied by normal x-rays. A suprapatellar bursal fat-blood level is sometimes the only sign of a fx. Patellar fxs not visible on standard views may be further studied with *oblique* or *skyline* views. A radiolucent gap

>2mm between a total knee prosthesis and bone is consistent with prosthetic loosening.

Ankle/hindfoot - A true *mortise* view is best done without any casts, if possible. The joint space should be uniform all the way around and the talar dome intact. Any widening of the space is significant, and proximal fxs should also be ruled out. The figure on the right demonstrates widening of the medial joint space.

On *lateral* view, calcaneal and 5th metatarsal base fxs (e.g., avulsion fx related to the peroneus brevis tendinous attachment) may be noted. If a calcaneal fx is suspected (e.g., fall from a height), a *calcaneal axial* view can also be ordered, although most fxs will be seen on lateral views.

B. Selected Issues in Computed Tomography

IV contrast - Radiopaque iodinated contrast is absorbed into tissues with high blood perfusion and capillary leakage. For example, the blood-brain-barrier (BBB), when intact, minimizes contrast enhancement of the brain parenchyma. However, if the BBB is disrupted (e.g., tumor, infection), these areas will enhance with IV contrast.

Contraindications to IV contrast include allergy to the dye, renal insufficiency, pheochromocytoma, multiple myeloma, and sickle cell crisis.

Acute ischemic stroke - Noncontrast CT is the initial imaging study of choice in acute suspected stroke to rapidly differentiate nonhemorrhagic strokes from conditions that follow different tx pathways, e.g., hemorrhage or tumor. Contrast is *not* given since acute blood appears bright on a non-contrast CT, and the addition of IV contrast in vessels can be confused with subarachnoid hemorrhage.

Initial CTs in ischemic stroke are often grossly unremarkable, although subtle signs (e.g., effacement of gray-white matter borders) may be seen. After about 24 hrs, a poorly circumscribed hypodense area (±mass effect) corresponding to cytotoxic edema may be seen. During weeks 2-3 post-stroke, the edema will subside. The infarct may exhibit contrast enhancement during the subacute phase. In the chronic stage, the infarct may appear as a relatively well-delineated hypodensity or cystic cavity.

Spine - CT is generally preferable to MRI for evaluating fine cortical bony detail (e.g., fxs), spinal neuroforaminal stenosis by bony elements, and facet arthropathy. Although somewhat controversial, bony central cervical canal stenosis is probably best appreciated on CT. Lumbar stenosis is best evaluated by MRI. An AP canal diameter of <10-11.5mm in the adult cervical or lumbar spine is generally considered stenotic and often consistent with clinical syndromes. Some criteria are more stringent (<7mm). Although AP diameters are often mentioned, canal shape (e.g., round vs. trefoil), canal area, the presence of soft tissue elements (e.g., herniated disk fragments), and other factors can play a significant, if not more important, role in determining clinically significant stenosis.

C. Magnetic Resonance Imaging (MRI)

1. Principles, contraindications, and IV Gd contrast

MRI distinguishes tissue types by their relative fat and water content, among other factors. On *T1-weighted images*, fatty tissue is bright and water is dark. On *T2*, water is bright (mnemonic: T2 H2O), while fat is less bright. Generally speaking, T1 shows anatomic detail well, while T2 is useful for distinguishing normal from pathologic tissues.

Spin echo (SE) sequences are high-quality (↑signal to noise), but acquisition times can be lengthy (e.g., 15 min). *Gradient echo* (GRE) offers different advantages (e.g., faster, allows for thinner [<2mm] sections), but is more susceptible to artifact and generally lower in image quality.

Contraindications to MRI include cardiac pacemakers/ defibrillators, implanted neural stimulators, cochlear implants, metallic orbital foreign bodies, and ferromagnetic cerebral aneurysm clips. External fixation devices are relative contraindications (may cause local burns).

IV gadolinium (Gd) contrast has paramagnetic properties and enhances the signal from well-vascularized or edematous tissues (e.g., viable tumor) on T1. Gd is often used with *fat suppression* techniques to reduce signals from fat, which may obscure areas of interest due to its brightness on T1. Gd images should be compared with non-contrast studies. Moderately severe reactions to Gd (e.g., laryngospasm, urticaria, tachycardia) are rare compared to CT contrast reactions, occurring ~1/5000.[1] *Relative contraindications* to Gd include hemolytic anemia and impaired renal function (e.g., CrCl <20 mL/min, depending on institution).

References: **1. Goldstein HA**: Safety assessment of gadopentetate dimeglumine in US clinical trials. *Radiology* 1990;174:17-23.

2. Selected clinical applications

Ischemic cerebral stroke - The infarcted area may begin to appear hyperintense on T2 SE starting ~6-12hrs post-stroke, although this window may vary. Subacutely, infarct signal may be high on T2, although in some cases, it may be difficult to visualize w/o IV Gd. In the chronic stage, the lesion may be high signal with better demarcated borders on T2, low signal on T1, and non-enhancing with Gd.

Diffusion-weighted imaging (DWI) is useful in acute ischemic stroke, particularly in differentiating newer strokes (e.g., w/in the last ~20days) versus older strokes. New lesions on DWI are visible within 2hrs and are exceptionally ("light bulb") bright, almost exclusively representing areas of irreversible ischemia. Old lesions arc poorly demonstrable on DWI.

Spine, spinal cord - A degenerated intervertebral disk has reduced signal intensity and vertical height compared to an intact disk on T2. Anular tears can produce a high signal focus that may enhance with Gd. Disk herniations are hypointense (relative to a normal disk) on T2 and may be recognized by their epidural fat displacement on T1. Disk degeneration, bulges, and herniations, however, are often seen in asymptomatic adults, increasing in frequency with age[1]. In the postoperative spine, IV Gd can help distinguish recurrent disc herniation from postoperative fibrosis.

An axial T1 or fast SE T2 sequence can be useful in assessing lumbar spinal canal size and facet joints. Compression of the thecal sac or nerve roots can also be evaluated on T2. Compressed nerve roots may have ↑ signals and enhance with Gd due to a local inflammatory response.

Metastatic spinal disease typically involves multiple vertebrae, is hypointense on T1 and hyperintense on T2, and enhances with Gd. *Short tau inversion recovery* (STIR) is a fat suppression sequence that can improve contrast between normal bone and metastatic lesions. Osteoporotic fxs are typically isointense and tend to lose Gd enhancement with time.

Acute spinal cord contusion and edema appear bright on T2, but remain fairly isointense to the cord on T1. In the chronic stage, myelomalacia (composed of scar tissue, microcysts, and degenerated neural elements) is hypointense to the cord on T1 and bright on T2. Spinal cord cysts are dark on T1 and bright on T2. Arachnoiditis may enhance on postcontrast T1.

Acute cord hematomas are typically hypointense on T1 and bright on T2. Subacutely, cord hematomas may become hyperintense on T1, before returning to a hypointense appearance as the clot becomes chronic.

Miscellaneous neurologic - Neurologic consultation and MRI may be indicated in the evaluation of *headaches* with certain worrisome features (e.g., persistently focal or exertional h/a; association with seizure, mental status change, or focal neurologic signs).

Multiple sclerosis plaques are bright on T2, and intermediate to dark (typically non-visualized) on T1. The *fluid attenuated inversion recovery* (FLAIR) sequence can improve plaque visualization. Gd can help to differentiate acute (enhancing) versus chronic (non-enhancing) plaques.

In *acute inflammatory demyelinating polyradiculoneuropathy*, Gd will brightly enhance the roots.

Musculoskeletal - Indications for musculoskeletal MRI include assessment of the severity and extent of injury; obtaining an expedient diagnosis in order to initiate prompt treatment; and ruling out soft tissue masses. Selected common applications follow.

Shoulder - An intact, uninflamed supraspinatus tendon is typically dark on T1 and T2. The "magic angle" artifact is a mildly increased signal in the middle portion of a non-pathologic tendon on T1. Coronal and oblique T2 sections demonstrating high signal in a non-retracted tendon suggest a partial-thickness tear. Evidence of a complete tear includes retracted tendons, filling of the void with high-signal fluid accumulation, and atrophy of the muscle. MR arthography with intraarticular (IA) Gd is the most sensitive and specific study in detecting rotator cuff tears[2], and is very useful when the diagnosis is equivocal. IA Gd is also useful in the evaluation of the glenoid labrum and glenohumeral ligaments.

Findings seen in classic extrinsic impingement syndrome can include an anteriorly hooked or low-lying acromion, subacromial enthesophyte, and thick coracoacromial ligament.

References: **1. Boden S**: Abnormal MR scans of the lumbar spine in asymptomatic subjects. *JBJS Am* 1990;72:403-8. **2. Tirman PFJ**: A practical approach to imaging of the shoulder with emphasis on MRI. In Boutin RD, ed.: Musculoskeletal Imaging Update. *Orthopedics Clinics of North America* 1997;28:483-515.

Knee - An intact ACL appears as a hypointense linear band on T2. Signs consistent with a tear include non-visualization of the ACL, hyperintense signal w/in the ACL, and a wavy appearance of the fibers.

Normal, intact menisci appear as triangular structures on sagittal views, and are hypointense on all sequences. Acute traumatic tears are typically hyperintense and vertically oriented and extend to the meniscal surface. Degenerative meniscal lesions can also be hyperintense, but are typically horizontally oriented and may not extend to the meniscal surface.

Advanced/research applications - *Functional MRI* uses the magnetic properties of blood to make realtime movies of blood flow changes (e.g., in the brain) as pts are exposed to various stimuli or perform tasks and so on.

MR spectroscopy (MRS) can quantify tissue concentrations of biochemical compounds noninvasively. For example, ↑ choline levels and ↓ *N*-acetylaspartate (NAA) correlate with demyelination and can detect lesions (e.g., MS) occult to conventional MRI. ↓ NAA may be a relatively specific measure of axonal injury and is investigationally being used to quantify damage in neurologic injury. High lactate levels correlate with hypoxia.

D. Triple-Phase Bone Scan (BS)

The triple-phase BS detects gamma radiation from short-lived radiotracer isotopes (e.g., 99m-technetium) that accumulate in areas of high bone turnover (e.g., tumor, fracture, trauma, infection, arthritis, and biomechanical stress). The **3 phases** are the 1) *blood flow* phase (centered on the body part of interest); 2) static *blood pool* phase (soft tissues); and 3) static *bone* phase (taken ~3hrs post-tracer injection). A "4th phase" (~24hrs) is sometimes used to assess suspected osteomyelitis in the distal skeleton of pts with poor peripheral circulation (e.g., diabetic foot ulcer).

Findings on BS are generally highly sensitive but poorly specific. BS, for example, detects heterotopic ossification (HO) and osteomyelitis ≥ 1wk before the x-ray. BS can also detect small fxs, nondisplaced fxs, compression fxs, and stress fxs missed by and before plain x-ray.

Despite low specificity, BS can be useful in appropriate cases for refining the differential diagnosis or guiding management. For example, a *tibial stress fx* can be positive in all 3 phases and will usually appear as a round, focused lesion, whereas *medial tibial stress syndrome* (shin splints) will be negative in the flow and pool phases but appear as a long, vertical, diffuse lesion in the bone phase. In the diagnostic w/u of *complex regional pain syndrome*, the blood flow and pool phases may show asymmetric uptake, while the bone phase (the most sensitive phase) shows increased periarticular uptake. In *acute back pain*, certain lesions noted on other studies (e.g., compression fxs or spondylolysis), can be differentiated as acute ("hot" on BS and potentially related to the current pain) versus chronic ("cold" and possibly not the direct cause of pain). In *HO*, hyperemia and ongoing increased bone phase activity are signs of HO immaturity and suggest to clinicians that surgical excision may be premature.

In some clinical scenarios (e.g., diabetic foot ulcer), BS is combined with *radiotracer-labeled WBC* scans in an attempt to improve specificity.

XXI. Pharmaceuticals

A. Selected Common "Rehab Drugs"

Note - **The following doses are for adults**. *Contraindications* always include hypersensitivity to the drug itself. *"Warn/Prec"* are some warnings that should be made and conditions where the medication may impose additional risk of adverse reaction. "Most common" side effects may be marked with an asterisk. The information presented here is obviously abridged; please refer to the PDR or product inserts for more information, including pediatric dosing guidelines.

alendronate (Fosamax, Merck) - [tabs 5, 10, 35, 40, 70mg] *Indic/ Dosage*: osteoporosis prevention: 5mg qd or 35mg qwk; osteoporosis tx: 10mg qd or 70mg qwk; Paget's disease: 40mg qd x6 months; all tabs should be taken ≥30 min before 1st food or beverage of the day, with a full glass of water; avoid lying down for at least 30 min; *Action*: biphosphonates act to inhibit normal and abnormal bone resorption; as a result, an asymptomatic reduction in serum Ca and PO_4 is noted; *Contra*: hypocalcemia, severe renal dysfunction, dysphagia; *Warn/Prec*: upper GI disease, pregnancy C; *Adverse Rxs*: esophagitis, GI distress, h/a, myalgias, arthralgias, back pain, dysphagia, abdominal distension, chest pain, peripheral edema, flu-like symptoms, esophageal ulcer.

amantadine (Symmetrel, Endo) - [cap 100mg, syrup 50mg/5mL] *Indic/Dosage*: Parkinson's disease/syndrome: 100mg bid, can increase to 400mg/d after one or several wks, start at 100mg qd for those on other anti-Parkinson's meds or medically ill pts; tx or prophylaxis for influenza A: 200mg initially, then 100mg qd; off-label for poor arousal or inattention in TBI: 100mg bid; off-label for post polio syndrome pain, fatigue in MS, and hyperthermia of central origin in TBI; *Action*: blocks ions channels (nicotinic ACh, M2 ionic channel in influenza A); also believed to release dopamine from intact dopaminergic terminals; *Warn/Prec*: seizure disorder, CHF, renal disease, pregnancy C; withdrawal from amantadine should be gradual; *Adverse Rxs*: (usually well tolerated) dizziness*, nausea*, nervousness, ataxia, insomnia, dry mouth, GI hypomotility, urinary retention, changes in mood, confusion, hallucinations, CHF, edema, orthostatic hypotension, livedo reticularis (particularly women).

amitriptyline (Elavil, Merck) - [tabs 10, 25, 50, 75, 100, 150mg] *Indic/Dosage*: depression: 50-150mg qhs (for elderly 10mg tid and 20mg qhs may be sufficient; reduce dose for hepatic impairment); off-label for neuropathic pain (start at lower doses than for depression); *Action*: tertiary amine tricyclic, NE/serotonin reuptake inhibitor; also has anti α1-adrenergic and potent antimuscarinic properties; may potentiate analgesic effect of opiods; *Contra*: acute post-MI, concomitant MAOI use; *Warn/Prec*: CV disorders (can cause HTN), hyperthyroidism, schizophrenia/paranoia, pregnancy D, d/c before elective surgery; withdraw gradually after long-term use to avoid insomnia and abdominal discomfort; *Adverse Rxs*: dry mouth*, blurred vision*, constipation*, urinary retention*, cardiovascular effects (tachycardia*, prolongation of AV conduction), weight gain, somnolence, seizures, photosensitivity, GI distress, leukopenia, gynecomastia, testicular swelling, sexual dysfunction, menstrual irregularity; *Monitoring*: baseline and periodic leukocyte and differential counts, LFTs, ECG. Pts with cardiovascular issues require surveillance.

baclofen (Lioresal, Novartis) - [tabs 10, 20mg, intrathecal] *Indic/ Dosage*: spasticity: titrate to max dose of 20mg qid as follows: 5mg tid x3d, then 10mg tid x3d, then 15mg tid x3d, then 20mg tid x3d, increase as needed; consider IT if oral effective but titration limited by side-effects; no indication of oral form for spasticity due to stroke, Parkinson's disease, or CP; *Action*: analogue of γ-aminobutyric acid thought to bind to GABA-B receptors, inhibiting Ca influx into presynaptic terminals and suppressing spinal cord excitatory neurotransmitters; *Warn/Prec*: impaired renal function, risk of seizure if withdrawn too quickly (therefore, should taper off over ~1wk), pregnancy C; *Adverse Rxs (oral baclofen)*: drowsiness*, dizziness*, h/a*, N/V*, lassitude*, GI upset*, urinary frequency, CNS depression, confusion, slurred speech, nasal congestion, seizures, blurred vision, weakness, hypotonia, HTN, CV collapse, respiratory failure, rash, pruritus, increased LFTs; *(IT baclofen)*: fatigue*, drowsiness*; *Overdosage*: IV physostigmine 1-2mg. Also see p.112 for details on IT baclofen.

capsaicin (Zostrix, Medicis) - [cream 0.025%, 0.075%, both OTC] *Indic/Dosage*: FDA approved for postherpetic neuralgia; commonly used for OA and neuropathic pain: apply a thin film to affected areas tid to qid; may require ongoing use for effect; experimental intravesical instillation inhibits contractions in neurogenic bladders; *Action*: evidence suggests capsaicin depletes the pain neurotransmitter substance P from unmyelinated peripheral neurons; *Warn/Prec*: wash hands after application, avoid contact with eyes, avoid heating pads in treated areas; *Adverse Rxs*: local burning sensation*, which typically improves with repeated use, but may not be tolerated by some.

carbamazepine (Tegretol, Novartis) - [tabs 100, 200mg, XR (bid) tabs 100, 200, 300, 400mg, oral susp 100mg/5mL] *Indic/Dosage*: epilepsy: start at 200mg bid; trigeminal neuralgia: start 100mg qd; off-label for neuropathic pain: start at 100mg bid; max dose for all indications is 1200mg/d, usually divided in tid doses, increase doses each wk by ≤200mg/d; *Action*: unknown, but related to the TCAs; may be a result of Na channel blockade in rapidly firing neurons and reduced excitatory synaptic transmission in the trigeminal nucleus; *Contra*: TCA hypersensitivity, h/o bone marrow depression, concomitant use of MAOIs (or w/in 14d of d/c); *Warn/ Prec*: impaired liver/renal fxn, hyponatremia, pregnancy C, numerous drug interactions; *Adverse Rxs*: (initially: dizziness*, ataxia*, drowsiness*, N/V*, but usually subside spontaneously w/in a wk), bone marrow suppression, hepato/nephrotoxicity, nystagmus, rash, Stevens-Johnson syndrome, arrhythmias; *Monitoring*: pre-tx CBC, BUN, LFTs, Fe, with periodic f/u (frequency guidelines not established).

celecoxib (Celebrex, Pfizer/Searle/Pharmacia) [caps 100, 200mg] *Indic/Dosage*: OA: 200mg qd or 100mg bid; RA: 100-200mg bid; acute pain/dysmenorrhea: 400mg initially, followed by 200mg if needed on first day, then 200mg bid prn; *Action*: COX-2 selective NSAID; *Contra*: hypersensitivity to sulfonamides, ASA, NSAIDs; *Warn/Prec*: HTN, CHF, h/o GI bleed, renal insufficiency; monitor INRs closely with concomitant warfarin tx, pregnancy C, nasal polyps; *Adverse Rxs*: edema, GI distress/bleed, thrombocytopenia, nephro/hepatotoxicity, bronchospasm, agranulocytosis. *Note*: In the

CLASS study (Silverstein FE: Celecoxib Long-term Arthritis Safety Study. *JAMA* 2000;284:1247-55), annual incidence of upper GI ulcer complications (bleeding, perforation, obstruction) for celecoxib 200mg bid vs. NSAIDs (ibuprofen 800mg tid or diclofenac 75mg bid) was 0.76% vs 1.45%; when combined with symptomatic ulcers, annual incidence was 2.08% vs. 3.54% (p=0.02).

clonidine (Catapres, Boehringer Ingelheim) - [tabs 0.1, 0.2, 0.3mg, TTS qwk patch 0.1/24, 0.2/24, 0.3mg/24hr] *Indic/Dosage*: HTN: start orally at 0.1-0.3mg bid, or TTS 0.1mg/24hr qwk, maximum dose is 2.4mg/d orally or TTS 0.3mg/24hr qwk; off label for spasticity: dosing similar to HTN; IT clonidine used investigationally for spasticity and neuropathic pain; *Action*: central α-adrenergic agonist that ↓ sympathetic discharge; *Warn/Prec*: CV disease, impaired liver/renal fxn, withdraw gradually to avoid rebound HTN, pregnancy C; *Adverse Rxs*: dry mouth/eyes, h/a, dizziness, nausea, constipation, sedation, weakness, fatigue, orthostatic hypotension, edema, anorexia, erectile dysfunction, joint pain, leg cramps.

cyclobenzaprine (Flexeril, Merck) - [tab 10mg] *Indic/Dosage*: muscle spasm due to acute painful musculoskeletal conditions: 10mg tid, max 60mg/d, not to exceed 2-3wks; *Action*: structurally related to the TCAs; thought to act on the brainstem to reduce skeletal muscle hyperactivity, but not effective for spasticity of central origin; *Contra*: TCA hypersensitivity, concomitant MAOIs (or w/in 14d of d/c), recovery from acute MI, CHF, arrhythmias, conduction disturbances, hyperthyroidism; *Warn/Prec*: glaucoma, prostatic hypertrophy, pregnancy B; *Adverse Rxs*: drowsiness*, dizziness*, dry mouth*, weakness, taste changes, fatigue, parathesias, nausea, insomnia, blurred vision, seizures, hepatitis, tachycardia.

diazepam (Valium, Roche) - [tabs 2, 5, 10mg, oral soln 5mg/5mL, 5gm/1mL, injection] *Indic/Dosage*: skeletal muscle spasticity due to local reflex spasm, UMN spasticity, athetosis, stiff-man syndrome: 2-10mg po/IM tid-qid (geriatric pt, 1-2.5mg qd-bid); anxiety dosing similar to spasticity; EtOH withdrawal: initially 2-5mg IV, repeat q3-4hr prn; status epilepticus: 0.2-0.5 mg/kg/dose IV q15-30min to a max of 30mg; *Action*: proposed mechanism for antispasticity effect is a post-synaptic facilitation of spinal cord GABA w/o a direct GABA-mimetic effect; *Contra*: CNS depression, acute angle glaucoma; *Warn/Prec*: class IV, impaired liver/renal fxn, depression may worsen with use, pregnancy D; *Adverse Rxs*: sedation*, "hangover"*, dizziness*, ataxia*, diplopia, hypotension, confusion, constipation, urinary retention/incontinence, anterograde amnesia, dependency, withdrawal syndrome, bone marrow suppression, rash, fever, hepatotoxicity, blood dyscrasias, injection site reaction (local pain and thrombophlebitis); apnea/cardiac arrest (rare, typically only after IV administration or in elderly or medically ill pts).

dantrolene (Dantrium, Proctor & Gamble) - [caps 25, 50, 100mg, injection] *Indic/Dosage*: spasticity: start 25mg qd, increase by 25mg q4-7d to max of 400mg/d divided bid-qid (considered the oral agent of choice in TBI due to peripheral action and less CNS side effects); off-label for malignant hyperthermia: 2mg/kg IV push until symptoms subside or cumulative dose of 10mg/kg reached; also off-label for heat stroke and cocaine overdose rigidity; *Action*: reduces excitation-contraction coupling via reduction of sarcoplasmic reticulum Ca release; *Contra*: active liver disease, lactation; *Warn/ Prec*: risk of hepatic dysfunction higher in women or if >35y/o, cardiomyopathy or pulmonary disease present, pregnancy C; *Adverse Rxs*: weakness*, malaise*, sedation*, dizziness*, nausea*, diarrhea*, acne-like rash, pruritus, h/a, insomnia, photosensitivity, fatal/nonfatal hepatotoxicity (most commonly 3-12mos after initiation of tx, most cases resolve with d/c), seizures; *Monitoring*: baseline/periodic LFTs.

etidronate (Didronel, Proctor & Gamble) - [tabs 200, 400mg] *Indic/ Dosage*: Paget's disease: 5-10mg/kg qd, not to exceed 6mos, or 11-20mg/kg qd, not to exceed 3mos; HO w/ SCI: 20mg/kg qd x 2wks, then 10mg/kg qd x10wks; HO w/ THR: 20mg/kg qd x1mo pre-op, 20mg/kg qd x3mos post-op; *Action*: as with other biphosphonates, it inhibits hydroxyapatite crystal growth by preventing precipitation of soluble amorphous $CaPO_4$; also slows osteoblastic and osteoclastic activity; *Contra*: renal impairment; *Warn/Prec*: CHF, enterocolitis, long bone fracture, pregnancy C; *Adverse Rxs*: N/V*, GI distress, osteomalacia/inhibition of bone mineralization, fractures, bone pain, seizures, angioedema, stomatitis.

gabapentin (Neurontin, ParkeDavis) - [caps 100, 300, 400mg, tabs 600, 800mg, soln 50mg/mL] *Indic/Dosage*: partial seizures with or w/o 2° generalization: 300mg qhs on day#1, 300mg bid on day#2, 300mg tid on day#3, continue to titrate as tolerated to effect, up to 3600mg/d; off-label for neuropathic pain: similar dosing; off-label 2nd line tx for spasticity (see p.110); *Action*: unknown; a GABA analogue w/o activity at GABA receptors; hypothesized to alter the concentration or metabolism of cerebral amino acids; *Warn/Prec*: impaired renal fxn, pregnancy C; d/c gradually over 1wk (no known drug interactions); *Adverse Rxs*: (initially): somnolence*, dizziness*, ataxia*, but these usually resolve w/in 2wks of starting drug), fatigue*, nystagmus*, tremor, diplopia, nausea, nervousness, dysarthria, weight gain, leukopenia, thrombocytopenia, dyspepsia, depression, periorbital edema, myalgias.

lidocaine patch (Lidoderm, Endo) - [patch 5% (10x14cm)] *Indic/ Dosage*: FDA approved in 1999 to tx postherpetic neuralgia: apply ≤3 patches on intact skin over the most symptomatic area qd (12hrs on/12hrs off); off-label for other types of neuropathic pain; *Action*: diffusion of lidocaine into the local epidermis/dermis is thought to block conduction of impulses (inhibits Ca-mediated Na and K ion fluxes) and stabilize neuronal membranes; provides direct local analgesia w/o complete anesthetic block; *Warn/Prec*: do not reuse patches; avoid showers/swimming with patch on; when used appropriately, mean peak serum levels due to systemic absorption may reach about one-tenth the therapeutic level used for antiarrhythmia (these patches are safe); caution in pts with hepatic failure or on anti-arrhythmics; pregnancy B; *Adverse Rxs*: initially, local erythema, edema, and or parasthesias, usually mild and resolve w/in minutes to 1hr.

metaxalone (Skelaxin, Carnick) - [tab 400mg] *Indic/Dosage*: relief of discomfort associated with acute, painful musculoskeletal conditions: 800mg tid-qid; *Action*: not established, but may be due to general CNS depression; no direct action on contractile mechanism of striated muscle, motor end plate, or nerve fiber; *Contra*: h/o anemias, significantly impaired renal/hepatic fxn; *Warn/P rec*: liver impairment, pregnancy (unknown); *Adverse Rxs*: drowsiness, paradoxic CNS excitation, nervousness, N/V, irritability, dizziness, rash, leukopenia, hemolytic anemia, jaundice.

methylphenidate (Ritalin, Novartis) – [tabs 5, 10, 20mg] *Indic/ Dosage*: ADHD; narcolepsy; off-label for depression (as a stimulant) in elderly, cancer, and post-stroke: 10-15mg/d up to 40-60mg/d in 2-3 divided doses, typically 30-45mins before meals; *Action*: a mild CNS stimulant with action similar to amphetamines (believed to facilitate NE and dopamine release); *Contra*: glaucoma, Tourette's syndrome, severe anxiety, agitation; *Warn/Prec*: class II, HTN, seizure disorder, CV disease, numerous drug interactions, pregnancy C; *Adverse Rxs*: nervousness*, insomnia*, anorexia, h/a, dizziness, dyskinesia, rash, HTN, tachycardia, palpitations, GI distress, dependency, leukopenia, exfoliative dermatitis, erythema multiforme, motor tics, elevated LFTs, ventricular arrhythmias, thrombocytopenia.

modafinil (Provigil, Cephalon) - [tab 100, 200mg] *Indic/Dosage*: FDA approved in 1998 for excessive daytime sleepiness (EDS) due to narcolepsy: 200mg qd, 100mg in liver impairment; off-label for fatigue due to MS and to improve alertness post-TBI; being studied in Alzheimer's disease, age-related memory decline, and EDS due to sleep and neurologic disorders; *Action*: thought to act on the anterior hypothalamus and other CNS centers; increases glutamatergic while reducing GABAergic transmission; *Contra*: cardiac disease; *Warn/Prec*: class IV, impaired liver/renal fxn, pregnancy C; *Adverse Rxs*: headache*, nausea*, infection* (2° to decreased immune fxn due to sleep reduction), nervousness*, anxiety*, insomnia*, rhinitis, diarrhea, dry mouth, anorexia, dizziness, depression; *Monitoring*: consider periodic LFTs.

oxybutynin (Ditropan, Alza) – [tab 5mg, oral susp 5mg/5mL] *Indic/ Dosage*: bladder instability: 5mg bid-tid, max 5mg qid; *Action*: muscarinic blocker with a direct antispasmodic effect on smooth muscle; *Contra*: myasthenia gravis, GI obstruction, ileus, ulcerative colitis, megacolon, obstructive uropathy, glaucoma; *Warn/Prec*: impaired liver/renal fxn, pregnancy B; *Adverse Rxs*: dry mouth*, nausea*, blurred vision*, tachycardia*, flushing*, decreased sweating, dry eyes, constipation, urinary retention, dizziness, drowsiness, insomnia, hallucinations, restlessness, cycloplegia, erectile dysfunction.

phenytoin (Dilantin, ParkeDavis) – [caps 30, 50, 100mg, XR caps 30, 100mg, chewable tabs 50mg, oral susp 125mg/5mL, injection] *Indic/Dosage*: epilepsy: start 100mg po tid, max 600mg/d to therapeutic levels of 10-20mcg/mL (may load orally with 1g given as 400mg, 300mg, 300mg separated by 2hrs each, then start regular dosing 24hrs after load); status epilepticus: load with 10-15mg/kg IV slowly, followed by 100mg oral/IV q6-8hrs; *Action*: centrally acting modifier of Na, Ca, K ion transport that results in membrane "stability"; blocks Na channels in a use-dependent manner; *Contra*: sinus bradycardia, SA block, 2nd/3rd degree AV block, Adams-Stokes syndrome; *Warn/Prec*: hypotension, CV disease,

DM, impaired liver/renal fxn, arrhythmias; thyroid disease, pregnancy D, porphyria, elderly; *Adverse Rxs*: anorexia*, dyspepsia*, nausea*, ataxia*, nystagmus, diplopia, lethargy, insomnia, constipation, tremor, slurred speech, h/a, rash, blood dyscrasias, megaloblastic anemia, severe dermatologic rxns, hepatotoxicity, severe CV abnormalities, purple glove syndrome, toxic delirium, lymphoma, SLE, gingival hyperplasia, coarse facies, osteomalacia; *Monitoring*: trough level should be drawn after 1wk of regular use to determine steady state level; draw level 2-4hrs after IV loading dose; no strict guidelines for drawing levels after oral loading.

prednisone - [tabs 1, 2.5, 5, 10, 20, 50mg, oral soln 5mg/5mL] *Indic/Dosage*: inflammatory disorders: 5-60mg qd; *Action*: adrenocorticosteroid with glucocorticoid and mineralocorticoid activity; *Contra*: systemic fungal infection; *Warn/Prec*: seizure disorder, osteoporosis, CHF, DM, HTN, TB, impaired liver fxn, pregnancy C; *Adverse Rxs*: edema, mood swings, psychosis, adrenal insufficiency, immunosuppression, peptic ulcer, CHF, insomnia, anxiety, hypokalemia, osteoporosis, appetite change, h/a, dizziness, HTN, hyperglycemia, acne, cushingoid features, skin atrophy, ecchymosis, impaired wound healing, menstrual irregularities.

rofecoxib (Vioxx, Merck) - [tabs 12.5, 25, 50mg, susp 12.5mg/5mL, 25mg/5mL] *Indic/Dosage*: OA: 12.5-25mg qd; acute pain/dysmenorrhea: 50mg qd ≤ 5 days; *Action*: COX-2 selective NSAID; *Contra*: hypersensitivity to ASA, NSAIDs; *Warn/Prec*: HTN, CHF, h/o GI bleed, renal insufficiency, monitor INRs closely with concomitant warfarin tx, pregnancy C, nasal polyps; *Adverse Rxs*: edema, GI distress/bleed, thrombocytopenia, nephro/hepatotoxicity, bronchospasm, agranulocytosis.

sildenafil (Viagra, Pfizer) - [tabs 25, 50, 100mg] *Indic/Dosage*: Erectile dysfunction: start at 50mg about 1hr prior to sexual activity, increase up to 100mg or decrease to 25mg as needed; 25mg recommended for age >65; *Action*: selective PDE-5 inhibitor that increases cGMP levels and promotes smooth muscle relaxation in the corpus cavernosum; *Contra*: regular or intermittent nitrate use (may result in death due to severe hypotension), MI/stroke w/in 6mos; *Warn/Prec*: liver/renal disease, hypotension, penile deformities, seek medical attention for erections >4hrs, no nitrates for cardiac events or autonomic dysreflexia for 24hrs after sildenafil ingestion; *Adverse Rxs*: h/a*, flushing*, dyspepsia*, nasal congestion*, visual problems* (blurred vision, blue tinge, photophobia), priapism, UTI, diarrhea, dizziness, hypotension, tachycardia, MI, TIAs, stroke.

tizanidine (Zanaflex, Elan) - [tab 4mg] *Indic/Dosage*: spasticity: no set dosing; sample regimen: start 2mg qhs, then q3d increase to: 2mg qam/2mg qhs→2mg qam/4mg qhs→ until 4mg tid is achieved; maximum dose is 36mg/d; *Action*: central α-2 adrenergic agonist that reduces spasticity by increasing presynaptic inhibition of motoneurons; reportedly ~10% of the BP effects of clonidine; peak effects at 1-2hrs after administration; *Warn/Prec*: impaired renal/hepatic fxn, pregnancy C; *Adverse Rxs*: somnolence*, weakness*, hypotension, dry mouth, dizziness, hepatotoxicity, severe bradycardia, hallucinations, asthenia, UTI, constipation, urinary frequency, flu-like symptoms, pharyngitis, rhinitis, increased spasms.

tolterodine (Detrol, Pharmacia) - [tabs 1, 2mg, LA tabs 2, 4mg] *Indic/Dosage*: bladder instability: 2mg bid, 1mg bid in hepatic dysfunction; (with Detrol LA, 2 or 4mg qd); *Action*: muscarinic blocker that exerts a direct antispasmodic effect on smooth muscle; *Contra*: narrow-angle glaucoma, gastric or urinary retention; *Warn/ Prec*: impaired liver/renal fxn, pregnancy C; *Adverse Rxs*: dry mouth*, blurred vision*, dry eyes*, urinary retention, UTI, somnolence, h/a, dizziness, GI distress, URI, flu-like symptoms, arthralgia, pruritus.

topiramate (Topamax, Johnson & Johnson/Ortho-McNeil) - [tab 25, 100, 200mg, cap 15, 25mg] *Indic/Dosage*: FDA approved in 1997 as an adjunct tx for partial onset seizures and mood stabilizer: start at 25mg bid and increase daily dose 50mg/wk until therapeutic (typically 200-400mg/day); Ortho-McNeil pursuing indication for diabetic neuropathy (initial J&J studies not promising); off-label use for neuropathic pain: no established dosing regimen, may start at 25mg qhs with weekly increases of 25mg/day; clinical trial to study possible slowing of ALS progression in progress; *Action*: Na channel blocker, but analgesic mechanisms unclear; *Warn/Prec*: pregnancy C; *Adverse Rxs*: somnolence*, dizziness*, vision problems*, unsteadiness*, nausea, parasthesias, psychomotor slowing, nervousness, speech/memory problems, tremor, confusion.

tramadol (Ultram, Johnson & Johnson/Ortho-McNeil) - [tab 50mg] *Indic/Dosage*: FDA approved 1993 for moderate to moderately severe pain: 50-100mg q4-6hrs, not to exceed 400mg/day (elderly: ≤300mg/day; creatinine clearance <30mL/min: dose q12hrs, ≤200mg/day; hepatic impairment: 50mg q12hrs); one 50-mg tab is roughly equivalent to one Tylenol #3; *Action*: centrally acting, synthetic non-opioid analogue of codeine that produces analgesia by weak μ-receptor agonism (has 10% of the affinity of codeine), serotonin/NE reuptake blockade, and enhancement of neuronal serotonin release; opioid-like CNS side-effects, and thus may be better tolerated in injured workers who wish to remain working; *Contra*: acute EtOH intox; use with opioids, psychotropics or central analgesics; *Warn/Prec*: seizure disorder, head trauma, increased ICP, concomitant MAOI or SSRI, pregnancy C, acute abdominal conditions, opioid dependence; *Adverse Rxs*: vertigo*, nausea*, constipation, h/a, somnolence, vomiting, pruritus, asthenia, sweating, dry mouth, dyspepsia, diarrhea, syncope, orthostatic hypotension, tachycardia.

trazodone (Desyrel, Apothecon) - [tabs 50, 100, 150, 300mg] *Indic/ Dosage*: depression: 150-400mg in divided doses; off-label for aggressive behavior: 50mg bid, titrate prn; take with food to enhance bioavailability; *Action*: triazolopyridine derivative antidepressant; mechanism not fully understood (serotonin reuptake inhibitor in animal models); *Contra*: early post-MI period, pregnancy C; *Warn/ Prec*: CV disorders, nursing, d/c before elective surgery; *Adverse Rxs*: drowsiness*, N/V*, dizziness, dry mouth, constipation, urinary retention, hypotension, bitter taste, fatigue, blurred vision, h/a, arthralgia, incoordination, tremor, priapism (~1:6,000-10,000).

B. Sample Dosing of Selected Oral NSAIDs

diclofenac (Voltaren) - [tab 25, 50, 75mg] 50-75mg bid; Voltaren XR [tab 100mg] 100-200mg qd; Arthrotec (diclofenac/misoprostol) 50-75mg/200 bid or 50mg/200 tid.

etodolac (Lodine, Ultradol) - [tab 200, 300, 400mg] 200-400mg po bid/tid; Lodine XL [tab 400, 500, 600mg] 400-1200mg qd.

ketoprofen (Orudis) - [tab 25, 50, 75mg] 25-75mg tid/qid.

ketorolac (Toradol) - 15-30mg IV/IM q6hr or [tab 10mg] 10mg po q4-6hr; total duration of ketorolac treatment not to exceed 5days.

meloxicam (Mobic) - [tab 7.5mg] 7.5-15mg qd.

nabumetone (Relafen) - [tab 500, 750mg] 1000-2000mg qd or 500-1000mg bid.

naproxen (Naprosyn, Aleve) - [tab 250, 375, 500mg] 250-500mg bid.

oxaprozin (Daypro) - [cap 600mg] 1200mg qd.

C. Opioids

Morphine-like narcotic agonists have activity at the μ and κ opioid receptors, and possibly the δ receptors. The μ receptors mediate supraspinal analgesia, euphoria, respiratory and physical depression, miosis, and reduced GI motility. The κ receptors mediate spinal analgesia, sedation, and miosis. Unlike NSAIDs, which have a ceiling effect for anesthesia, opioids act in a dose-dependent manner and can control all intensities of pain with increasing doses up to the point of surgical anesthesia. The major drawback is side effects, which are also dose-dependent.

Equianalgesic Dosing Table[1]

Medication	Equianalgesic IM/IV	PO	T1/2	Dur	Sample Initial Dosing
codeine	120	300	3h	4-6h	15-60mg po q4-6h
fentanyl (Duragesic Patch)	100µg	—	—	—	25µg/hr patch, q3days
hydrocodone (Lortab,Vicodin)	—	30	—	4-6h	various products/ dosing
hydromorphone (Dilaudid)	1.5	7.5	2-3h	4-6h	2-4mg po q4-6h
meperidine (Demerol)	75	300	3-4h	4-5h	75-150mg IV/ IM q3-4h
methadone (Dolophine)	—	20	—	6-8h	various dosing
morphine	10	30	2-4h	4-6h	10-30mg po q4h
morphine CR (MS Contin)	—	30	—	8-12h	15mg po q8-12h
oxycodone	—	30 PO 15 PR	—	3.5h	5-10mg po q4h
oxycodone CR (Oxycontin)	—	30	—	8-12h	10-40mg po q12h
pentazocine (Talwin)	60	180	2-3h	4-6h	30mg IV/IM q3-4h

All dosing above in **mg** except where noted. The dosing table should be used as follows: to convert from drug A to B, calculate the total # of mg of drug A given over a 24hr period. Convert total to drug B using the columns under "equianalgesic" above. Administer that amount of drug B over 24hrs.

Reference: **1.** Loeser J, ed.: *Bonica's Management of Pain*. 3rd ed. LWW. 2000.

D. Injectable Corticosteroids

	hydro-cortisone	predni-solone	methyl-prednisolone	triam-cinolone	beta-methasone
relative potency	1	4	5	5	25
onset	fast	fast	slow	moderate	fast
duration of action	short	intermediate	intermediate	intermediate	long

Sample steroid/analgesic injections

Shoulder bursitis/rotator cuff tendinitis (lateral approach) - Using a 1.5" 21-gauge needle, inject a 5mL mix of 20mg triamcinolone and local anesthetic to the lateral shoulder 2cm anterior and inferior to the acromial angle at a depth of ~2cm below the skin.

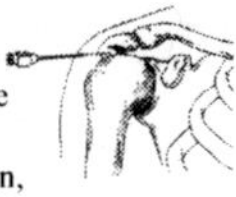

Lateral epicondylitis - Rest arm on a table palm down, elbow flexed 45°. Using a 1.5" 23-gauge needle, inject a 5mL mix of 10mg triamcinolone and local anesthetic into the most tender area about the extensor tendon attachment to the lateral epicondyle.

Fig.1

Carpal tunnel - Supinate the wrist and extend over a towel. Using a 1.5" 25-gauge needle, inject a 1mL mix of 10mg triamcinolone and local anesthetic directed distally at a 60° angle to the skin proximal to the distal wrist crease between the palmaris longus and FCR tendons. The needle is inserted 1-2cm. Median n. anesthesia confirms proper injection; paresthesias may last 1-2 wks. Volume is minimized to reduce post-injection discomfort.

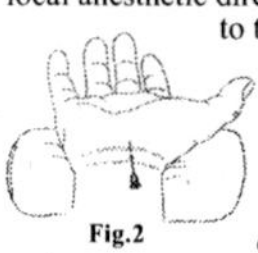

Fig.2

DeQuervain's tenosynovitis - Place the forearm on a table on its ulnar side in ulnar deviation (support under the distal forearm with towels). Using a 1" 25-gauge needle, slowly inject a 5mL mix of 40mg triamcinolone and local anesthetic at a 45° angle along the APL and EPB sheaths to create a sausage-like wheal. If resistance is encountered, retract the needle to avoid tendinous injection.

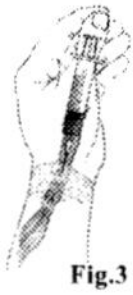

Knee - Seat the pt with knees flexed 90° and the feet dangling. Using a 1.5" 21-gauge needle, inject a 5-6mL mix of 20-40mg triamcinolone and local anesthetic either medially or laterally to the patellar tendon towards the intercondylar notch. Discourage excessive post-injection ambulation x24hrs.

Fig.3

Pes anserine bursa - With the pt supine and knee in extension, advance a 1.5" 21-gauge needle perpendicularly to periosteum at the point of max tenderness (medial leg), then pull back slightly. Inject a 4mL mix of 20mg triamcinolone and local anesthetic.

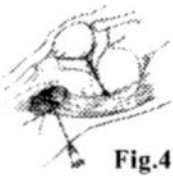

Fig.4

Plantar fascia - Place pt prone on a table w/ feet extending over edge. Advance a 1.5" 23-gauge needle at the point of maximal tenderness near the medial attachment of the plantar fascia to calcaneus. Retract ~2mm from the periosteum and inject a 2mL mix of 20-40mg triamcinolone and local anesthetic.

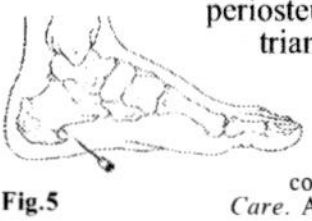

Fig.5

Figs.1,2,4,5 courtesy of **Steinbrocker O**, ed.: *Aspiration and Injection Therapy in Arthritis and Musculoskeletal Disorders.* Harper & Row, 1972. **Fig.3** courtesy of **Snider RK**, ed.: *Essentials of Musculoskeletal Care.* American Academy of Orthopaedic Surgeons, 1997.

XXII. EMERGENCIES

A. Management of Acute Autonomic Dysreflexia (AD)

1. Immediately **raise the head of the bed or sit the pt upright** if supine (to reduce cerebral hyperperfusion). Loosen clothing and devices. Quickly survey for precipitating causes, beginning with the urinary system. If there is an indwelling catheter, remove kinks and twists and check for correct placement. If there is no catheter, premedicate the urethra with 2% lidocaine jelly and **catheterize** the bladder. Check BPs frequently, e.g., q2-5mins.

2. If no relief and SBP remains ≥150mm Hg (this value for adults has been determined by expert consensus; it may be lower for children and adolescents[1]), consider one of the following agents:

a. **Nifedipine** (Procardia) 10mg immediate release, using the bite-and-swallow (or puncture-and-swallow) technique (*not sublingually*). May repeat in 30mins. Use with caution in the elderly or with CAD.
b. **Nitroglycerin** (NTG)*, e.g., 1" of 2% NTG ointment† (Nitrobid), applied above the SCI level; or sublingual NTG (e.g., 0.4mg).
c. Other options may include (with sample doses): *amyl nitrate* 1 ampule inhaled; *hydralazine hydrochloride* 10mg IM/IV, push over 30secs; *clonidine* 0.1-0.2mg po; *prazosin* 1-2mg po; or *captopril* 25mg po.

3. If **fecal** impaction is suspected, liberally apply lidocaine jelly into the rectum. Wait 5mins, then gently disimpact. If AD worsens, discontinue disimpaction, insert more jelly and wait ~20mins before resuming.

4. Other potential sources of noxious stimuli include UTIs, cystitis, high fecal impaction, pressure ulcers, cellulitis, detrussor dyssynergia, HO, deep or superficial thrombophlebitis, ingrown toenails, trauma, diverticulitis, cholecystitis, appendicitis, GI bleeding/perforation, infectious or gouty arthritis, nephrolithiasis, endometriosis, epididymitis, ischemia, vaginitis, ovarian rupture, testicular torsion, or pulmonary infarct.

5. Observe pt and check BPs for ≥2hrs after resolution. If AD does *not* resolve, consider need for *intensive care* (if untreated, acute AD may lead to stroke or seizure). Consider need for *chronic antihypertensive therapy*, e.g., ACE inhibitors, terazosin, clonidine, transdermal or oral nitrates, or β-blockers.

B. Anaphylaxis[2]

Tx - *Epinephrine* 0.3-0.5mg sc (0.3-0.5mL of a 1:1000 soln), repeat ~q20min prn. If there is major airway compromise or hypotension, prepare to *intubate* and consider 0.5mL of 1:1000 epinephrine soln sublingually, or 3-5mL of 1:10000 soln IV/ET tube. An IV drip titrated to BP may be necessary for the most severe rxns. *Antihistamines*, which relieve skin symptoms and shorten rxn duration, may be useful adjuncts. Observe for ≥6-8hrs because symptoms may recur after resolution of the initial episode. *Steroids* (e.g., methylprednisolone 125mg IV or hydrocortisone 500mg IV) have limited immediate effects, but may ↓ the likelihood of early relapse.

---

*Avoid with recent (<24hrs) sildenafil intake. † Advantageous because of quick removal. References: **1**. *Clinical Practice Guideline: Acute Management of AD: Individuals with SCI Presenting to Health-Care Facilities*, 2nd ed. Consortium for Spinal Cord Medicine, 2001. **2**. *The Washington Manual of Medical Therapeutics*, 29th ed. LWW, 1998.

INDEX